Herb Antivirals

Basics, Recipes and Natual Remedies for Emerging and Resistant Viral Infections

Naili FK

Table of Contents

Introduction

Congratulations on purchasing *Herb Antivirals,* and thank you for doing so.

The chapters following this introduction will discuss what herbal antivirals are and just how easy it is to use them to make you well and keep yourself healthy. The idea of using herbs as medicine has been around since time began. There were hundreds of years when the only available medications when a person was sick were the herbs that the local shaman, healer, priest, or medicine man made available to the patient. These herbal healers studied the herbs they used, studied their effectiveness in different forms, and whether or not they actually worked on sick people. These healers also grew or gathered their own herbs and processed them for their own use.

Using herbal concoctions for medication became less popular with the advent of the pharmaceutical medication. It became so easy to take a pill for whatever ailment the patient was suffering from. People kept themselves healthy on a poor diet by taking copious amounts of vitamin pills. While the modern world left herbals behind, the underdeveloped areas of the world continued to use them, since pharmaceuticals were scarce, and if they were available, the cost was prohibitive.

People soon noticed that the residents of these other countries were somehow healthier, and they lived longer, more satisfying lives than many people did in developed countries. People wanted to know what the secret was. The secret for these people came from nature, in the form of herbs that had been used for centuries to make people well and keep people healthy. These same herbs that were once used only by the local healer suddenly found new fame as everyone wanted to live a life free from chemicals and other unhealthy ingredients.

Viruses are here to stay. But with the help of herbal antivirals, we can keep ourselves healthier and lessen the effects of any viruses if we should catch one. This book will provide you with all of the information that you need to begin using your own antivirals to ward off disease in your life and make your body strong and resistant to viruses. Using herbs to fight viruses is not a new idea, but it is slowly regaining favor in the world. With the information in this book, you will be one of those people who are ready to move forward into healing yourself.

There are many books on this subject on the market today, so thanks to you again for choosing this one! All efforts were made to ensure that it is full of as much useful information as possible, so read on, and please enjoy!

Chapter 1: The History of Herbals and Antivirals

The Ancient World of Herbs

Herbs have healing properties that have not changed very much in the last five thousand years. If a healing herb that was available then is still available today, then it will have the same ability to heal now as it did then. In ancient times the people who used herbs for their healing powers spent a great deal of time gathering the herbs, growing the herbs, preparing the herbs, and studying the herbs. Even before journals were kept outlining the power of the individual herbs, healers kept this information safely tucked away in their minds, and they passed this information down to family members and other healers.

Humans have always been fascinated with the flowers and plants that inhabit the world in which we live. The oldest records of written folklore regarding plants and herbs come from ancient Egypt. Their medicine was used along with magic to heal people. Many people believed that magic was the main ingredient in the healing of the sick person, where the magic was most likely the healing powers of the herbs that were used. In India, herbs are often used in religious and medical practice to make people well and keep them healthy. In the Far East, it was common practice to use the petals of flowers to make healthy teas from. When trade opened between the Far East and the rest of the world sailors brought back knowledge of different uses for herbs, along with the herbs they returned with. At that time, many of the herbs in use were still being used along with magic for healing. People who lived then were still used to the idea that magic was the real healer, and the herbs were just things that the healer used when conducting their rituals. Eventually, the partnership between magic and herbs was disconnected, and many people began studying the herbs and learning all there was to know about them.

During the Middle Ages, herbs already had many everyday uses. They were used to season and preserve food. People who did not bathe regularly would carry herbs to mask the smell of their persons. Herbs were used for dyeing and tanning leather, and for coloring other types of cloths. During this time, the only medicines that were available were created from herbs since pharmaceutical medications had not yet been developed. The monasteries in Europe preserved the studies of herbalism. Monks would grow gardens full of useful and common medicinal herbs, as well as spending time each day in the study and translation of the works of the ancient Greeks and Romans who wrote about herbs and their properties.

At the end of the Middle Ages, learned men began to change the idea of science from something speculative to a process of experimentation. This was the beginning of the separation between medical and biological science and the tradition of herbalism. Those herbalists who moved into the scientific circle began to identify and classify herbs, a study that gave rise to the science of botany. They worked alongside doctors and scientists to study the uses of different herbs and created scientific medicine.

At this time, medicines began changing. At that time, the idea of medicine was still rooted in the use of herbs. Teas, soups, poultices, and tinctures were made from fresh or dried herbs and mixed with alcohol or water to create a remedy for an illness or a preventive against illnesses. Much of medical science was still ruled by the two prevailing ideas of treatment at the time, the doctrine of signatures or the doctrine of humors. The doctrine of signatures referred to the idea that nature made specific herbs to treat ailments in specific areas of the body. The herb lungwort has leaves that are shaped like the lobe of a lung, so it was considered to be a good remedy for lung diseases. The doctrine of humors stated that the liquids that were inside of the body – the black bile, yellow bile, phlegm, and blood – needed to be kept healthy so that the person would be kept healthy. Certain herbs were used for the treatment of ailments of certain humor in the body. While more and more medical doctors populated the earth, many of them still used herbal medicines in their practice. Patients were accepting of this because the doctor was at least trying to heal them.

The Industrial Revolution in the latter half of the nineteenth century brought about many technological developments and ignited the development of the technological side of medicine. People became more interested in homeopathy, where individuals would take the toxic ingredients that doctors were using and dilute them or add extra ingredients to them. These were then used for the same cures that doctors used them for, but in a new, lower dose that would not risk killing the patient. Scientists began experimenting with making powders and pills from herbs and chemicals, potions designed to combat illnesses. Based on the knowledge of the herbs, scientists actually did create three authentic drugs that could be used to heal people of their illnesses: cocaine, digitalis, and quinine. This launched the modern era of medicine. Shortly after that, aspirin was developed, and medicine moved from a world of herbal remedies into one where a patient could take a pill and feel almost instant relief from their illness. Never mind that these new drugs all came from some sort of herbal concoction; people wanted quick and convenient medications. They wanted a pill or a liquid that would cure them instantly, or as quickly as possible.

How Viruses Spread

The word 'virus' is often used, where it should not be used. Many people attribute a minor feeling of illness to having been caused by a virus. If your stomach is queasy, then you must have caught a virus. If you are sneezing and coughing, then you must have caught a virus. Some of these symptoms are caused by viruses, that is true, but not every bad physical feeling is the result of a virus.

A virus is an organism that is even tinier than a bacterium. It is made up of human DNA or RNA, the genetic material that makes us the people that we are with the characteristics that we have. This genetic material carries around many different types of diseases. These diseases range in severity from the common cold and the influenza virus to the more serious ones like Acquired Immunodeficiency Syndrome (AIDS) and Human Immunodeficiency Virus (HIV). When a virus enters your body, it uses its genetic material to change your cells or to cause damage inside of you to give the virus the ability to rapidly multiply. Most times, people are able to fight off a virus by simply resting and hydrating themselves until the virus runs its course and dies out. When people are not strong enough because of pre-existing illnesses or age, then the virus might be fatal to them.

Viruses are spread between humans in various ways. They type of virus that it si will determine how it is spread. A virus can be spread through coughing, sneezing, sharing needles, sexual contact, or by some sort of oral transmission. When people touch other people or touch surfaces that someone has coughed or sneezed on, and then they touch their eyes, nose, or mouth, they run the risk of transmitting a virus to themselves. This is usually how the common cold spreads from person to person. The flu virus (influenza) is mostly spread through respiratory droplets, such as are expelled when someone sneezes or coughs.

Measles is transmitted through the air since the particles of the virus stay suspended in the air for several hours after the infected person sneezes or coughs.

The more serious viruses, the AIDS or HIV or Hepatitis B viruses, require that two people share blood, bodily fluids, or have direct sexual contact with each other. HPV (human papillomavirus) and herpes can be transmitted from one person to another through hand holding or kissing. Sometimes viruses will live for a short time period on an inanimate object like a doorknob, a countertop, or a used tissue.

Some viruses are transmitted from animals to humans through the raw meat of the animal. When people prepare the meat, and either do not cook it to the proper temperature or they contaminate work surfaces with the blood of the meat, they run the risk of spreading these viruses. The meat does not need to actively bleed on a surface to leave traces of blood too small for the human eye to see. And humans can transmit human viruses to other people when they prepare foods without washing their hands first.

Other than completely avoiding contact with other people, it is impossible to completely avoid being around viruses. The best ways to avoid getting sick with a virus is to wash your hands, avoid touching your face, and staying in general good health.

Modern Uses for Herbal Remedies

Herbal remedies have been a significant part of our culture and history as long as there has been culture and history. No matter where your ancestors lived, they most likely used herbs for medicinal and dietary purposes. As people experimented with more plants and learned more about various plants, they committed this knowledge to memory and passed it down to their descendants. There is currently a renewed interest in herbal medicine as people look for ways to move away from pharmaceutical medicines and on to more natural remedies. In herbal medicine, the value of the plants and their individual parts, the flowers, seeds, leaves, bark, stems, and roots, are all used and respected. Modern medicine was born on the foundation of herbs being drunk as restorative teas, mixed into salves for skin irritations, and ground into powders for a hundred other uses. Herbal medicine started the history of what is known as modern medicine. Current medicinal uses for herbs are found most often in homeopathic medicine and aromatherapy. Homeopathy is the practice of using herbs to cause physical reactions that mimic the illness the patient has to spur the body to want to heal itself. Aromatherapy involves the use of essential oils that have been derived from herbs to create strong odors that cause a sense of well being in the patient and induce healing.

While the Romans and Greeks probably started the use of herbs as medicine, the Chinese and the people of India keep the practice alive even today. Traditional Chinese Medicine is built on the belief that the health of the human is based on keeping balance internally since the internal forces of yin and yang are always battling for control. When they are balanced, through healthy living and herbal medicines, the person remains healthy. Ayurvedic medicine from India is still a very popular practice even today. It also stresses the idea of living life in balance with the use of proper diet and herbal medicines.

Herbal remedies are probably just as popular today as they were five thousand years ago. They are available in many different forms, from liquids, capsules, powdered, chopped, and dried. They can be swallowed as pills, added to your bathwater, rubbed on the skin in a lotion or cream, or brewed and drunk as a tea. Today's herbal supplements are considered to be food items and not drugs, and so are not closely regulated by any government agency. But while herbal supplements are not standardized and regulated, they are also not ever referred to as a cure for a specific illness. The label might say that a particular herb will enhance your mood, but it is not allowed to say that the herb will relieve your depression.

There are safe ways to use herbal supplements to relieve the symptoms of an illness or to help strengthen your immune system. If you are already taking a prescription for something, then it is best to consult with your doctor or pharmacist, since some herbs and some medications can interact unfavorably together. But if you are in reasonably good health and you have done your research on the benefits of a particular herb and its possible side effects, then there is no reason to not use herbs to supplement other measures you are taking to ensure your continued good health.

Chapter 2: Forms of Herbal Medicine

Herbal medicine is also known as botanical medicine or herbalism. It is a system of medicine that is based on the use of plants or the different parts of plants.

Herbal medicine has been used since ancient times to assist bodily functions and treat illnesses. One of the best ways to take advantage of the healing powers of herbs is to use their ability to prevent disease. There is an herb that will treat or prevent nearly every ailment that humans suffer from. Herbs work in a way that is similar to many of the pharmaceutical preparations currently available because herbs contain many types of naturally occurring chemicals. Many of the pharmaceutical medicines still in use today are still derived from plants.

Morphine, the pain medication, is derived from the opium poppy, and quinine, which is used to treat malaria, comes from the bark of the cinchona tree.

To make sure that the balance of chemicals in the plant are fully utilized, many herbalists believe that the herbs should be used in their complete form. Many herbalists believe that the herb is best utilized when it is used to treat ongoing, chronic conditions. Just like with pharmaceutical medicines, there are no herbs that will perform a quick fix for any ailment. Remedies that are made out of herbs come in a wide variety of forms and may be used for external or internal applications.

Teas, Infusions, and Decoctions

Three of the most common ways in which people use herbs for medicinal purposes are when they make teas, infusions, or decoctions. Teas are made by pouring boiling water over an herb and letting it sit for up to five minutes, to bring the flavor of the herb into the tea. The herb is then discarded. An infusion is a stronger form of a tea, where the boiling water is poured over the herb and then the entire mass is left to sit and steep or brew for a longer period of time to make the concentration of the herb stronger in the water. A decoction is an infusion that has been reduced by half. This method makes the concentration of the herb in the water even stronger, as you would find in herbal syrup. To make a decoction, you will first make an infusion, and then you will allow the infusion to simmer over a low heat while the steam evaporates. This will make the liquid much more concentrated. You can easily do this process at home. Set a pot of infusion on the stove over a medium to high heat. As the infusion warms, the steam will begin to float off of it. When this happens turn the heat under the pot down so that the liquid will continue to simmer while steam continues to rise off of the infusion. When about half of the liquid has evaporated then strain the liquid to remove the herb and you will have a decoction. Store this liquid in a glass bottle and keep it in a dark place until you need to use it.

You make an infusion to be able to release more of the nutrients, vitamins, minerals, and chlorophyll from the herb than you would be able to release when making tea. This is the reason why infusions are considered to be medicinal remedies. Besides making an elixir that is more concentrated than simple tea, the infusion will allow you to extract the medicinal properties from stems or bark because these will need more processing than you will be able to get from tea. You can easily make an infusion at home by placing one cup of any dried herb into boiling water in a quart jar. Put the lid securely on the jar and let it stand for at least four hours. You can make the infusion in the evening and let it sit overnight to provide you with a strong morning tea. When the infusion has soaked for the right amount of time, strain out the herbs, and then squeeze the water out of them to put it back into the infusion. An infusion can be kept in the refrigerator for up to three days, and you would either drink it cold or heat it for a strong flavored tea. When steeping parts of herbs and plants for an infusion or to make a decoction and you want the best results then you will need to steep seeds and berries for at least thirty minutes, flowers and flower petals for at least two hours, leaves for four hours minimum, and roots and barks will need at least four hours.

Herbal tea is a very easy and versatile drink to make and a very good way to make use of the healing properties of different herbs. When you make tea, you will brew the dried or chopped fresh herbs in boiling water for at least five minutes.

Only a tiny amount of herb is used for making tea and you will not get too much medicinal value from teas. Herbal teas are often referred to as tisanes. If the tea is being prepared for a medicinal purpose, it is usually for an upset stomach, a headache, or to soothe the symptoms of a cold or respiratory illness. Try one of these recipes for a delicious and nutritious antiviral herbal tea.

Evening Tea for Nourishment

Ingredients:

- One teaspoon of dried Lemon Balm leaves before they flower
- One cup of water
- One half teaspoon of dried Holy Basil leaves and flowers
- One half teaspoon of dried nettle leaves

Directions:

1. This tea can easily be made from fresh varieties of the listed ingredients if you prefer to use fresh herbs since they will make the taste stronger. The recipe using dried herbs will give a nurturing, comforting, woodsy taste where the fresh herbs will give a lively sparkling flavor.
2. Place the fresh or dried herbs in a large teacup or bowl and pour the hot water over them to cover them completely.
3. Let the mixture steep for about ten minutes before straining out the herbs and drinking the tea.
4. This tea will provide many nutrients and is a good drink to drink after dinner to aid your digestion.

Fresh Fennel Tea for Settling the Stomach

Ingredients:

- One cup of hot water
- Sprig of peppermint
- Two tablespoons of fresh fennel frond

Directions:

1. Chop the fennel fronds into small pieces, cover them with the hot water, and steep the teas for about ten minutes.
2. The sprig of peppermint is added at the end for taste.
3. This tea is a good stomach relaxer, and drinking it regularly will help to provide protection against viruses that attack the stomach.

Congestion and Coughs Tea

Ingredients:

- Four cups of water
- One half cup of dried eucalyptus root pieces

Directions:

1. Put the eucalyptus roots in the four cups of water in a pot and let this soak for at least one hour, although overnight is better.
2. Then boil the mixture, and then cover the pot partially and reduce the heat.
3. Let this mix simmer for at least fifteen minutes before straining it and drinking.
4. This tea will help eliminate the viruses that cause colds and upper respiratory congestion.

Tea for Sore Throats and Head Congestion

Ingredients:

- Four cups of water
- One fourth cup of dried Marsh Mallow root pieces
- One fourth cup of dried honeysuckle
- Two tablespoons of dried eucalyptus leaf pieces
- One fourth cup of dried Marsh Mallow leaf pieces
- One tablespoon of dried licorice root pieces
- One tablespoon anise seeds lightly crushed

Directions:

1. Put the dried licorice, anise seeds, eucalyptus leaf, and the Marsh Mallow root pieces in a pot, cover them with the four cups of water, and bring this mixture to a boil.
2. Cover the pot partly and turn down the heat so the mixture will simmer for about twenty-five minutes.
3. Strain the herbs from the mix and let the liquid cool for five minutes.
4. While the liquid is cooling, put the honeysuckle flowers and the Marsh Mallow leaf into a teapot.
5. Pour the liquid from the roots over the flowers and let it steep for about five minutes before drinking.
6. This tea will help to fight the viruses that cause head and chest congestion.

Refreshing Iced Tea

Ingredients:

- Ten cups of cold water
- Two cups of ice cubes
- Fifteen sprigs of Salad Burnet
- Eight sprigs of Lemon Verbena, fresh

Directions:

1. Rinse the herbs well and chop them into small pieces.
2. Place the chopped herbs in a pitcher that will hold two quarts and cover them with the water.
3. Put the ice cubes on top of the herbs to help hold the herbs down in the water.
4. Let this mix sit for at least one hour in the refrigerator, although overnight is better.
5. This tea will have a sweet vanilla lemon flavor from the lemon verbena that will mix well with the tang of cucumber from the salad burnet. It can be made even sweeter by adding fresh stevia leaves.

Herbal Extracts (Tinctures)

A tincture is a herbal extract that is highly concentrated. They are made by soaking the roots, leaves (fresh or dried), berries, or bark of a plant in a solution of vinegar or alcohol. Soaking these in the vinegar or the alcohol will pull out the active ingredient from the parts of the plants and concentrate them in the liquid. Tinctures are made from one single plant or from a combination of plants. The species of plant being used will determine whether you use the berries, flowers, bark, roots, leaves, or the whole plant. Some tinctures should only be used externally, but many can be used internally.

It is very easy to make a tincture at home. You will first carefully sort the parts of the plant that you are using so that any parts that you don't want to use can be discarded. Chop the herbs coarsely before putting them in the liquid solution to help release the chemicals from the plant. Place the plants in the jar first and then cover them with the alcohol or the vinegar that you are using. Cap the jar tightly and let the solution sit for six to eight weeks. Once a day, you should shake the jar to help mix up the tincture and release more of the chemicals from the plants.

You can add more alcohol to the jar if the level seems to be dropping. When you feel the tincture has steeped for long enough just strain out the herbs and store the tincture in small glass bottles out of the light. Be sure to label the bottles so you will know what is in them.

Chamomile Tincture

Ingredients:

- Quart glass jar with lid
- One and three-fourths cups of vodka or rum
- One and three fourths cups of boiling water
- One cup of dried chamomile flowers

Directions:

1. Place the chamomile flowers in the glass quart jar.
2. Pour just enough boiling water over the flowers to cover them. You might need to stir the flowers gently to make sure they are all covered with the water.
3. Use the vodka to fill up the rest of the space in the jar. Put the lid on the jar and store it in a dark place for four weeks.
4. Remember to shake the jar once a day to mix up the ingredients.
5. After four weeks, strain the mixture through cheesecloth to remove all traces of the flowers.
6. Take one teaspoon in water to promote restful sleep.

Tincture for Digestion

Ingredients:

- Quart glass jar with lid
- One and one-half cups of vodka or rum
- One and one-half cups of boiling water
- One-fourth cup of dried fennel seeds
- One-half cup of very finely diced fresh ginger root
- One-half cup dried peppermint leaves

Directions:

1. Put the fennel, ginger, and the peppermint in the glass jar and cover them with the boiling water just until they are covered.
2. Use the vodka or the rum to fill up the rest of the jar. Place the lid on the jar and store the jar in a dark place for at least two, but no more than six weeks, shaking the jar daily.
3. After the mixture is done steeping strain it carefully and store the liquid in small jars.
4. Take one teaspoon in water as needed.

Echinacea Tincture

Ingredients:

- Pint size glass jar with lid
- One-half cup dried echinacea leaf
- Apple cider vinegar or rum or vodka
- Boiling water

Directions:

1. Fill the jar at half full with the echinacea leaf.
2. Pour the boiling water over the leaves just until they are moist.
3. Then fill the remainder of the jar with the vinegar or the alcohol and stir the mixture gently.
4. Put the lid on the jar and store it in a dark place for three to six weeks, remembering to shake it daily to mix the flavors.
5. Strain the liquid well and store the tincture in small jars.
6. Use a teaspoon in hot water to make a tea to soothe sore throats or colds.

Essential Oils

Essential oils are made by combining the compounds from the plant that hold the flavor and scent with oil to create an oil that has many different uses. When the chemicals have been extracted, they are then mixed with a carrier oil so that they can be used for medicinal or aromatherapy purposes. Essential oils are only used externally as they are not meant to be ingested. Many of the commercially available essential oils are not essential oils but infused oils, and the difference is very important. Infused oil is created by letting the herbs soak in oil so that some of the active compounds will be brought out of the plants. There are some herbs that will work quite well with using this method, but most herbs are better prepared as essential oils.

Essential oil is the essence of the plant oil in a concentrated form that is used for healing, among other things. Don't be confused by fragrance oils which are even weaker versions of infused oils and only carry the scent of the plant with none of its healing properties. There are two relatively easy methods that you can use to make your own essential oils at home.

Method One – With this method, you will be making the essential oil in a crockpot. You will need to gather together the pot, one or two gallons of distilled water, and enough of the fresh plant material, chopped roughly so that it will fill the crockpot halfway. Place the plant material in the crockpot and then pour in enough distilled water so that the crockpot will be three fourths of the way full. Set the lid on the crockpot but set it off to the side slightly so that the steam will be allowed to escape. Turn the crockpot on to high and leave it there until the water gets hot. When the water is hot turn the heat back down to low and let the mixture simmer for four hours. After four hours, the plant material will be cooked well. Turn off the crockpot and leave the mixture sitting there with the lid on until the mixture is cooled. When the liquid has cooled, set the pot part of the crockpot into the refrigerator and leave it there overnight. The next day, when you remove the crockpot from the refrigerator, there will be a thin layer of film on top of the water in the crockpot that will have hardened in the refrigerator.

Carefully remove the oil from the top of the water, but move as quickly as possible because it will begin to melt. Put the pieces of oil into a glass bottle and let it finish melting in a cool, dry place. This is the essential oil from the plant.

Don't forget to label the bottle before you store it away.

When you make essential oil this way, remember that plant material that is fresh will work much better than plant material that is dried out. Fresh plants will produce more oil than dried ones will. If you are harvesting plants from your own garden, try to harvest them first thing in the morning, after the dew has dried.

Make sure the plant is not carrying any bugs and do not use plants that are dead or diseased. This method will give you three to four teaspoons of essential oil.

Method Two – This method also uses four cups of roughly chopped plant material. Instead of using distilled water, you will use undenatured ethyl alcohol or unflavored vodka. For this application rubbing alcohol will not work. You will also need a large ceramic bowl or a ceramic crock. It must be ceramic; metal will not work. Put the herbs into the ceramic bowl and cover them completely with the liquid that you are using. Let the mixture sit undisturbed for twenty-four to forty-eight hours, covering the bowl with cheesecloth to keep out any dirt or insects that might get in. If you want to leave the mixture for longer than forty- eight hours, that is fine, because the longer that it sits the stronger that it will be. When you feel it has set long enough strain the herbs out of the mixture carefully. After the liquid has been drained off press the herbs so that you release any leftover oil that is in the herbs. Then put the liquid into the freezer and let it remain there overnight. The oil will rise to the top and freeze and you will be able to pick it off and store it in a glass bottle in a cool, dry place.

You will use essential oils to ingest, inhale, or to apply to your skin. They can be used in your bath, as a spray, in compresses, or to massage into your skin.

Essential oils are beneficial for treating breathing problems caused by viruses in the nose and chest. Simply place a few drops of an appropriate essential oil into a bowl of boiling water and inhale it to clear your congestion.

Creams (Balms)

A gentle but effective way to relieve ailments of the skin is with the use of salves and balms made from herbs. These can be purchased at any health store but they are also quite easy to make at home. There are three types of herbal topical treatments available to use. You can use infused oils or essential oils to soothe irritations of the skin. Lotions and creams mix together water and oil to make a soothing topical treatment. A salve is a solid combination of oil with soy wax or beeswax. The first step in making balms and salves is to make the essential oil.

These can be kept for up to a year after they are made.

To prepare an herbal salve, you will need to gather together the essential oil of your choice, clean metal containers or glass jars to store the salve in, a double boiler, one ounce of beeswax in either pellet form or grated, and eight ounces of infused herbal oil. Remember the infused oil and the essential oil are different things. Begin by warming the oil in the double boiler. If you do not have a double boiler, you will need to use two sauce pots, one smaller than the other so that it can sit inside the larger one. Put water in the larger pot, just a few inches, and set the smaller pot sown inside of the larger one. Put the oil in the smaller pot to warm it. When the oil is warmed, stir the beeswax into it, and keep stirring until all of the beeswax has been melted and mixed in well. When the beeswax is completely mixed in you can add a few drops of essential oil to add in scent. Pour the salve while it is still warm into the jars or tins that you are using to store it.

Put lids on the containers and store them in a cool, dark place. The salves will last for up to one year.

To make an herbal cream, you will need to gather together some clean glass jars with lids, an immersion blender or a regular blender, a double boiler, one half to one ounce of beeswax, three fourths cup of carrier oil like almond oil, one cup of rosewater or distilled water, and any essential oil for a scent that you might want to use. Mix the beeswax and the oil together in the double boiler and warm it on a low heat until the beeswax is completely melted. Pour the melted oil into the blender and let it sit and cool to room temperature. While the mixture is cooling, it will thicken and turn cloudy. When the mixture is properly cooled, blend it on a high speed and slowly add in the water while the wax is blending. If the blender seems to be getting hot just turn it off and let it sit for a few minutes. When the mixture becomes thick and turns white, then it is ready to use. You will now add in a few drops of essential oil for scent if you want to, but use no more than three drops and blend it in well. Put the cream into the glass jars, using a spatula to get all of the cream out of the blender. Put the lids on snugly and store the cream in a cool, dry place for no more than one month.

Soothing Eczema Balm

Ingredients:

- Fifteen drops thyme essential oil
- Fifteen drops cedarwood essential oil
- Twenty drops lavender essential oil
- One-fourth cup raw honey
- Two tablespoons almond oil
- Two tablespoons beeswax
- One-fourth cup shea butter
- One-half cup coconut oil

Directions:

1. Put the beeswax, shea butter, and the coconut oil in a quart glass jar.
2. Put two inches of water into a saucepan and bring it to a simmer, and then set the glass jar into the water.
3. Let it sit there until the ingredients have completely melted.
4. Take the jar out of the hot water and sit it off to the side to cool for five minutes.
5. Then add in the essential oils and the honey and stir everything together well.
6. Spoon the balm into a small glass jar with a lid and let it

completely cool.

7. Write the date on the jar and keep it for no more than one year.

8. This balm works great on skin issues.

Breathing Balm

Ingredients:

- One two-ounce glass jar
- Five drops of peppermint essential oil
- Eight drops of rosemary essential oil
- Ten drops of eucalyptus essential oil
- Thirteen drops of cypress essential oil
- One-fourth ounce of beeswax
- One-fourth cup of coconut oil or sunflower oil

Directions:

1. Put two inches of water into a double boiler and put the beeswax and the carrier oil in the top part.
2. Let it warm until the beeswax is completely melted and well mixed with the oil. Take this mixture off of the heat.
3. Put the essential oils into the glass jar and pour the beeswax oil mixture on top of them.
4. Place the lid securely on the jar and then shake it gently to mix all of the ingredients together well.
5. Let the jar sit undisturbed until the mixture has hardened, and then use it as a rub to ease stuffy breathing or muscle aches.

Antibacterial Salve

Ingredients:

- Ten drops of lavender essential oil
- Ten drops of tea tree oil
- One tablespoon of raw honey
- Four tablespoons of beeswax pellets
- One-third cup of dried calendula
- One-third cup of dried lavender
- One-half cup of coconut oil
- One-half cup of olive oil

Directions:

1. Blend the coconut oil and the olive oil in the top of a double boiler and warm it until the coconut oil is completely melted and well mixed with the olive oil.
2. Stir in the dried calendula and the dried lavender and let this simmer for thirty minutes.
3. Then strain the herbs out of the oil and put the oil back into the top of the double boiler.
4. Mix in the honey and the beeswax, stirring often until all ingredients are melted and well mixed.
5. Remove this from the heat and stir in the essential oils. Pour the mixture into a jar and put on the lid.
6. Let the jar sit for twenty minutes until the mixture is solid. Use this on skin irritations and scrapes.

Lavender Salve

Ingredients:

- One-fourth teaspoon lavender essential oil
- One-eighth teaspoon vitamin E oil
- One-half cup sweet almond oil
- One-fourth cup shea butter
- One fourth cup beeswax

Directions:

1. In the top of a double boiler, melt the shea butter and the beeswax until they are melted and well mixed together.
2. Stir in the sweet almond oil and let the mixture become liquid again.
3. Take this off the heat and let the mixture cool until it is down to one hundred thirty degrees.
4. Then stir in the essential oil and the vitamin E and pour the mixture into the containers.
5. Let it cool and become hard before putting the lid on the container.
6. Use this for skin irritations.

Herbal Compresses

There are many times in the life of the average person when an herbal compress might be needed. A cold in your chest, road rash from falling in the driveway, body aches from a weekend of gardening, or cramping in your muscles, any of these situations would benefit from the use of an herbal compress. This is one of the simplest herbal preparations to make because it usually involves nothing more than soft cloths and an herbal solution. Using an herbal compress will help to soothe inflammations and injuries and give the body the opportunity to calm down and heal itself. Depending on whether the compress used is cold or warm will depend on whether blood is forced away from the injured area or brought to it because either scenario can aid in healing.

Herbal compresses are relatively simple to make. They begin with a strong herbal decoction or infusion. You can also use herbal essential or infused oils for added scents if you like. All herbal compress remedies follow the same basic set of directions:

- Each cup of water you use will require three to four tablespoons of herbs
- If you are using hard plant material like berries, barks, or roots, then you will need to start by making a decoction first

- Add in any lighter plant materials that you might be using like flowers and leaves to the decoction when it is finished, putting a lid on it to keep the strength of the herbs in, and let it steep for thirty minutes
- If your compress will be using only lighter herbs like flowers or leaves, then cover them with boiling water in a glass bowl and put a lid over the bowl so that the steam will stay in while the mixture steeps for thirty minutes
- When the herbs have finished steeping strain them out of the water, using a cheesecloth to strain the water if the herbal compress is for injured skin
- Each cup of this infusion will need up to thirty drops of tincture
- Place a clean, soft cloth in the water and squeeze out the excess water, then apply the cloth to the injured or inflamed area
- If you are using a cold compress, let the mixture cool before using
- If you are using a hot compress reapply the compress when it cools, and reapply a cold compress when you can no longer feel the cooling relief

If you need to cover a large area or you might need to use the compress for several days, then feel free to make a large batch. You can keep the extra liquid in the refrigerator for up to two days. If the liquid is for a hot compress, then it can be warmed as necessary.

Cold compresses are great when you have pain with heat and inflammation like road rash, sore throat, bug bites, bruises, headaches, or minor burns like sunburns. A cold compress will ease the inflammation in the affected area by constricting the blood vessels to help soothe the area and start the healing process. A hot compress will ease the tension in the affected area by helping to bring blood to the area. The hot compress is good for congested lungs, sore throats, headaches, menstrual pain, muscle spasms, and pulled or strained muscles. When using a hot compress, it is important to make sure the compress is not so hot that it will burn the skin of the patient. Whichever compress you are using, it should be used for at least ten minutes at a time. To ensure complete relief, the compress should be used three or four times a day.

Chapter 3: Herbals to Boost Immunity

Your chances of catching a cold or the flu, or any of the other nasty little viruses that plague human beings, will be greatly lessened if your immune system is healthy and able to fight off intruders. You can easily achieve a healthy immune system by using natural methods to boost your immune system. Your immune system is your body's first line of defense against viruses. You will have a lower chance of becoming sick if your immune system is strong. Eating a well-balanced diet and getting the proper amount of sleep every night are important, but adding herbals into the mix will help to ensure that your immune system can fight off anything.

The primary goal of herbal medicine is to create inner strength by keeping the systems of the body working properly. This theory is practiced in Traditional Chinese Medicine and Ayurvedic medicine. The following eight herbs are some of the best herbs to use when you want to strengthen your immune system. They will help to bring balance to your body systems, boost your immune system, and bring you to an optimal level of overall health.

Medicinal mushrooms – Herbal medicinal practitioners in the Far East have used medicinal combinations of mushrooms for centuries to bring health and wellness to their patients. Medicinal mushrooms offer important health benefits. They will help you to fight off viruses, reduce inflammation, lower your cholesterol, and lower your blood pressure. They are also full of antioxidants that will keep your immune system healthy. There are four mushrooms in particular that are full of medicinal properties and antiviral goodness.

Lion's Mane – This is a globe-shaped snowy white fungus that is found growing on dying or dead broadleaf trees like the sycamore, maple, walnut, and oak. It is considered to be a gourmet mushroom that tastes something like eggplant. It is used to relieve the symptoms of people with gastric or esophageal cancers. It is effective against gastritis and several kinds of ulcers and helps to promote proper digestion. For your immune system, this mushroom will protect your gastrointestinal tract against the formation of tumors, inflammation, and various toxins from the environment.

Zhu Ling – This fungus comes in shades from white to grey and grows on the exposed roots of willows, beeches, maples, and birches or on dead stumps of trees. This mushroom helps to reduce the side effects of chemotherapy and is often used in the treatment of lung cancer. It can work to relieve the symptoms of chronic hepatitis. For your immune system, this mushroom will strengthen your white blood cells, increase the production of antibodies in your blood, and enhance and stimulate the overall performance of your immune system.

Reishi – This mushroom grows on the bark of various hardwood trees and comes in many different colors like black, purple, red, blue, yellow, and white. Although it is found all over the world, it is rare to find this mushroom growing in the wild, so most of the supply available now is grown and cultivated on commercial farms. Athletes use this mushroom to enhance the oxygenation of their blood, giving them more stamina, especially in areas of high altitudes. It is particularly good at preventing altitude sickness in people who regularly climb high mountains. It will reduce the thickness of your blood to make it flow easier through your arteries and veins. It will also help to lower your blood pressure and your cholesterol levels. For your immune system, this mushroom will enhance the performance of your white blood cells and help protect you against developing certain cancers.

Turkey Tails – This mushroom grows in large colonies in deep woods and comes in shades of red, blue, black, brown, gray, and white. It is shaped like the tail of a turkey, which is what gives this mushroom its name. This mushroom is highly effective when used against various cancers in combination with other medicines. It seems to lessen the negative side effects of cancer treatments while it enhances the power of the radiation treatments. It can also help to lower your blood cholesterol. For your immune system, this mushroom will provide powerful antioxidants that work to destroy free radicals. It also has powerful anti-viral properties and might even be effective in inhibiting the growth or the HIV virus.

Ginger – This root brings powerful decongestant and antihistamine properties. Ginger has been used in various forms of alternative and traditional medicine for centuries. Some of the more common uses for ginger are to lessen the effects of cold and flus, reduce nausea, and help with digestive ailments. You can use ginger powdered, dried, fresh, or in a juice or oil. It can treat various forms of nausea naturally, and it is particularly effective when used for morning sickness. Ginger has anti-inflammatory properties that help to reduce muscular aches and pains when it is taken daily. Extract of ginger, especially when taken with other herbs and spices, can help to relieve the negative effects of osteoarthritis, and it works whether it is taken orally or applied topically. When people who have type 2 diabetes use ginger daily, it can result in a decrease in their blood sugar levels.

People who have problems with chronic indigestion or other related digestive problems find relief when they use ginger in their cooking because it helps to empty the contents of the stomach faster, so it helps to move the food along and lessen the amount of time that it sits there digesting. Your blood cholesterol can be lowered if you take in ginger every day. And since the aging process is accelerated by chronic inflammation and oxidative stress, taking ginger daily or using it regularly in cooking can help to reduce the chance that you will developed those age-related diseases like cognitive decline and Alzheimer's disease. And ginger is very effective when used to eliminate or fight off infections since it is excellent at inhibiting the growth of many bacteria.

Andrographis – This is a plant that is common to the Far East and is regularly used for soothing sore throats, fevers, and digestive issues. It is a bitter-tasting herb that is full of compounds that give this herb antioxidant, antiviral, and anti- inflammatory properties. The underground stems and the leaves are used to make medicinal concoctions to treat and prevent the flu and the common cold. It is also used to treat a whole host of other physical ailments like indigestion, colic, gas, constipation, diarrhea, bronchitis, tonsillitis, sore throat, fever, and body aches. It is particularly effective for treating skin conditions like itchiness, ulcers, and wounds. It is also a potent astringent as it has both antibacterial and antiviral properties.

Elderberry – This fruit is native to North America and has been used in alternative and traditional medicine for centuries. There has recently been a renewed interest in the elderberry because it is loaded with minerals, vitamins, antioxidants, fiber, and other nutrients. The elderberry plant has been used throughout history, since the time of the ancient Greeks, to treat everything from cuts and burns to fevers and toothaches. All parts of the plant are safe to ingest after they have been cooked only; eaten raw, they can make you sick. Elderberry concoctions can be found in syrups, lozenges, pills, and powders. Elderberries help to encourage immunity and can lessen the effects of colds and flus. Elderberries contain powerful antioxidants that support the immune system. They will also enhance the immune response in the body by strengthening the proteins that carry messages for the immune system. Probably the biggest benefit the elderberry brings is the powerful antiviral agents it carries. Elderberries have a high concentration of chemicals that inhibit the ability of various viruses to attack the cells in your body.

Garlic – This amazing additive to foods is low in calories but high in vitamins and minerals. Garlic provides a wonderful boost of strength to your immune system. It can reduce the effects of the common cold and the flu. Regularly using garlic can help to lower your high blood pressure and your blood cholesterol levels. Lowering both of these will dramatically reduce the risk that you will develop heart disease. The antioxidants in garlic might help to prevent dementia and Alzheimer's disease. Because of all of these positive effects, regularly using garlic can help you to live longer. Garlic supplements can be used to enhance the performance of athletes. It can enhance the capacity to work hard and will also help to reduce fatigue. And garlic may be beneficial in preventing age-related bone loss and osteoporosis.

Honeysuckle Forsythia – This is not just a sweet-smelling flower on a pretty shrub. Honeysuckle forsythia is one of the fundamental herbs used in Traditional Chinese Medicine. This plant has impressive powers for eliminating toxins so it is particularly effective in treating skin issues like acne, abscesses, carbuncles, and boils. The entire plant, roots, fruits, stems, and leaves, can be used. Edible oils and good fats can be made from the seeds. You can use the leaves to treat sore throats, diarrheas, and high blood pressure. If you make a decoction of the fruits and flowers, you can use it daily to eliminate skin rashes, and it is especially gentle for face washing. Honeysuckle forsythia can relieve oiliness on skin, muscular inflammation, and vomiting.

Astragalus – This herb is an effective immune system booster. It is another one of the herbs that have long been used in Traditional Chinese Medicine. They use astragalus primarily to help treat cancer, cleanse the liver, and stimulate the immune system. The antiviral properties of this herb are especially beneficial in fighting viral infections like colds, flus, and hepatitis. It is also a potent antioxidant that will help to slow down the process of aging and deter many degenerative diseases. It will also provide health benefits to your lungs, circulatory system, and spleen. Astragalus is also useful for external applications since it is known to help heal wounds and improve circulation to wounded areas of the skin. And it is beneficial as a topical treatment for eczema, rosacea, and psoriasis.

Echinacea – This is a perennial herb that is native to North America and has been used by Native Americans for centuries. Echinacea contains potent active substances that are known to reduce inflammation and relieve pain. This plant has antioxidant and antiviral properties. The herb is often used to fight the common cold, particularly when it is drunk as a tea. It has the ability to inactivate the viruses that cause cold and flu. It is also effective against bacterial infections. Echinacea is also beneficial for those people who have compromised immune systems or those who are already fighting off a disease. Echinacea also works to fight off infections, inflammation, and various skin issues. It can enhance your mental health. And it can help to relieve the pain of various conditions like snake bites, sore throats, toothaches, and headaches.

Other Antiviral Herbs

In addition to the herbs that were already mentioned, there are several other herbs that have powerful antiviral properties, and most of them can be used every day in your kitchen for cooking.

Dandelion – While many people regard the dandelion as nothing more than a weed, but it does contain powerful antiviral agents. The leaves of the young dandelion plant are a great addition to a tossed salad and may inhibit the flu, HIV, and hepatitis B. Extract of dandelion may be a powerful treatment for dengue fever.

Ginseng – The root of this plant is widely used in Asian recipes and has long been used in Traditional Chinese Medicine. It is particularly effective at fighting off viruses. Studies have shown that ginger is significantly effective against hepatitis A, RSV, hepatitis B, the norovirus, the coxsackieviruses, and the herpes virus.

Licorice – This has been used in medicinal practice for many centuries. The active substances in licorice have potent antiviral properties that are effective against pneumonia, herpes virus, RSV, and HIV.

Rosemary – The oleanolic acid in this herb has antiviral properties that can work to inhibit hepatitis, the flu, HIV, and the herpes viruses.

Peppermint – This herb is often used to make tinctures, extracts, and teas that are often used to treat viral infections. The leaves produce oil that also has anti- inflammatory properties. Peppermint is particularly effective against viral infections of the lungs like bronchitis and RSV.

Lemon balm – This is a lemony plant that is often used in seasonings and teas. Its potent compounds have antiviral properties that can be used to fight HIV, bird flu, and the herpes viruses.

Fennel – This licorice-flavored herb is used in cooking vegetables and has properties that are used to fight viruses. It is particularly effective against viruses that cause respiratory infections, and it will also decrease inflammation and boost your immune system.

Basil – There are many varieties of this herb, and all of them contain antiviral properties. Sweet basil is effective against enterovirus, hepatitis B, and the herpes viruses. Holy basil can help to fight viral infections by boosting your immunity.

Sage – This aromatic herb has been used in alternative and traditional medicine for centuries to treat a variety of conditions. The stem and the leaves are particularly antiviral and may be used to inhibit HIV.

Oregano – This herb is very popular in cooking, especially in soups and casseroles, and it is also known for its antiviral properties. Oregano is useful against RSV, rotavirus, and herpes.

These herbs, and many more, are very easy to add to your daily routine by using them in recipes or in teas and compresses. Since they have powerful antiviral abilities, they should be regularly included in any way possible.

Chapter 4: Herbals to Fight Disease

Herbs and spices can be used to flavor foods, and they can also be used to fight diseases. Herbal remedies are plants that are used as medicines. They can be used to prevent disease or to cure diseases that already exist. Using herbs as medicines began in ancient times and continue today. The compounds in herbs that make them effective against diseases are the active ingredients of the herb. These herbs are among the best for their disease fighting properties.

Cinnamon – This herb was once considered to be more valuable than gold, and it was often used as a commodity for trade. Cinnamon will help to fight inflammation and mild pain. It also has amazing anti-aging properties.

Cinnamon is extracted by cutting the stems off of the cinnamon trees and removing the inner bark. This bark is allowed to dry, which makes it curl into cinnamon sticks. Cinnamon is full of antioxidants that will help protect your body from the damage caused by free radicals. It has anti-inflammatory properties that will repair damaged tissues and help your body fight infections. Regularly using cinnamon will lower your blood cholesterol and your blood pressure which may help to prevent heart disease. Cinnamon is also known to lower the levels of sugar in the blood so it may help to prevent or eliminate diabetes. One of the compounds in cinnamon helps to prevent the buildup of proteins in the brain which can lead to the development of Parkinson's disease and Alzheimer's disease. And regular consumption of cinnamon may help to prevent cancer.

Cloves – Cloves will relieve the pain of sore throats and toothaches. Cloves will stimulate the secretion of your digestive juices so that it will help to ease digestive issues. They are also good for relieving nausea, gas, and gastric irritability. Compounds in cloves have antibacterial properties that fight many human cancer, causing agents. In the early stages, cloves may be beneficial against lung cancer. The natural antioxidants in cloves help protect the body from free radicals, especially those that can cause damage to the liver. Since ancient times, cloves have been used as a natural medicine for diabetes. And cloves will help to keep your bones strong and healthy.

Ginkgo biloba – This antioxidant-rich herb will treat a variety of different conditions and can be used to enhance the health of your brain. Its use is popular in Traditional Chinese Medicine. The flavonoids in ginkgo biloba can protect against the diseases that are related to aging like dementia by increasing the flow of blood to the brain. This herb is also showing promise in the treatment of eye diseases like glaucoma. And the herb's ability to improve blood flow, especially to the eye, can help to reduce the incidence of retinal degeneration. Regular consumption may help to reduce blood pressure.

Turmeric – This warm, yellow-colored spice has an extensive history of use in traditional and alternative medicine. It comes from the roots of a flowering plant that is found in India and parts of Southeast Asia. Besides being delicious in foods and giving the bright yellow color to curry dishes, turmeric is known for its potent antioxidant and anti-inflammatory properties. Curcumin is the primary active ingredient in turmeric, and it is the compound that is responsible for the yellow color. Curcumin is what gives turmeric its health benefits. The major claim to fame that turmeric has is its ability to relieve pain by reducing inflammation in the body. It is speculated that in the proper doses, turmeric might be a better
anti-inflammatory treatment than over-the-counter medications that fight inflammation. Since chronic inflammation can contribute negatively to many chronic diseases, it is important to reduce the inflammation to help reduce the effects of the chronic illness or to eliminate it completely.

Turmeric helps to reduce high blood pressure, which can lead to strokes and heart attacks. It also helps to keep the muscles of your heart healthy which can help to reduce certain loss of function that is usually related to age, so it can reduce the likelihood that you will develop age-related heart problems. It is also effective in preventive related heart problems in people who have type 2 diabetes. And since excessive inflammation in the body is linked to the growth of tumors, the anti-inflammatory properties of turmeric may play a part in preventing and treating a wide variety of cancers such as gastric cancers, breast cancer, prostate cancer, pancreatic cancer, and cancers of the colorectal system.

People who suffer from osteoarthritis may find that turmeric is an effective and safe long-term option for treatment of the pain and stiffness that goes along with arthritis. Since turmeric is exceptional at relieving inflammation, it also helps to relieve the pain that swollen joints cause. Since turmeric can improve many of the contributing factors that lead to diabetes, this herb might also help to prevent high cholesterol levels in the blood, high blood sugar, and insulin resistance, which may help to eliminate or prevent type 2 diabetes.

Turmeric increases the levels of certain proteins in the spinal cord and brain that are responsible for keeping your nerve cells healthy and for regulating the communication between these nerve cells. This function is needed for memory and learning. Because of its ability to feed these beneficial proteins, turmeric may play an important role in preventing the onset of Alzheimer's disease. And the same proteins that play a role in Alzheimer's disease also play a role in depression. Turmeric is often found to be an effective antidepressant.

Rheumatoid arthritis sufferers may find relief when they use turmeric regularly. The anti-inflammatory properties of turmeric help with the inflammation that these arthritis victims suffer from. And turmeric also has amazing antimicrobial properties along with its antioxidant and anti-inflammatory properties, which make it an excellent defense against irritations of the skin. It is beneficial in the treatment of psoriasis, photo aging, eczema, and acne. The antioxidants in turmeric fight off the free radicals in your body that cause harm to all the cells in your body. It works by preventing particular enzymes from making specific free radical cells, it helps to control the enzymes that work to neutralize the free radicals, and it actually works to seek out and destroy many different forms of free radicals. And regular consumption of turmeric may help to prevent glaucoma.

Sage – Various cuisines around the world use sage to flavor their dishes since its earthy flavor and strong aroma lend heartiness and taste to almost any dish. It is a potent spice that can be used sparingly, and it is full of various nutrients and other healthy compounds. Sage is full of antioxidants that will strengthen your body's immune systems and help to neutralize free radicals that are harmful to your body and that may be linked to chronic diseases. In fact, sage contains over one hundred sixty distinct antioxidant compounds. It works to lower the bad cholesterol in your blood and improve your memory and the function of your brain.

Sage can neutralize the microbes that lead to the formation of dental plaque and cavities. It can also be used to fight mouth ulcers, infected gums, dental abscesses, and infections of the throat. The leaves of the sage plant can be brewed into a tea that is helpful for menstrual cramps. The sage extract will help to improve the body's sensitivity to insulin and will help to reduce blood sugar levels.

This herb works to prevent the breakdown of certain chemicals in the brain that promotes memory and brain function. And sage not only helps with memory but also with calmness, alertness, and helping to keep an elevated mood level. Sage not only stimulates the death of cancer cells but it also works t suppress the growth of new cancer cells. A traditional remedy for digestive upsets and diarrhea is fresh sage. Since it provides ten percent of the recommended daily allowance of vitamin K, it can help to keep your bones healthy. And certain compounds in sage may help to fight skin rashes and wrinkles.

Thyme – This herb is often overlooked in the kitchen because many people do not know what to do with it. But it is excellent for seasoning meats, poultry, and vegetables, as long as it is used in small amounts because it tends to be quite strong. But thyme has so many more uses that are not related to use in the kitchen. When fresh or dried thyme is steeped in vinegar or alcohol to create a tincture, it is effective when used against acne because of its antibacterial properties.

Regular consumption of thyme will help to reduce cholesterol and high blood pressure. Making tea with essential oil of thyme and hot water is good for soothing sore throats and relieving nagging coughs. And thyme is loaded with vitamin A and vitamin C, so it is an excellent herb to use if you feel a cold or other virus coming on.

Ginseng – Traditional Chinese Medicine has made use of ginseng for years. It is a short plant that grows slowly and is classified in one of three ways. It is called red, white, or fresh. If the ginseng is harvested after it has grown for six years, then it is referred to as red ginseng, ginseng that is harvested between four and six years of growth is called white ginseng, and any ginseng that is harvested before four years of growth is considered to be fresh. The most popular varieties of ginseng are Asian ginseng and American ginseng. They vary in the concentration of their active ingredients, so it is believed that Asian ginseng will have an invigorating effect on people, while American ginseng will have more of a calming effect.

Ginseng is loaded with anti-inflammatory and antioxidant properties. It is able to help improve mood, behavior, and memory as well as mental performance. The compounds in ginseng can help to strengthen the immune system. It also might assist in boosting the positive effects of basic immunizations, and it can help healthy people become more resistant to infections, particularly after surgery.

And because it works to reduce inflammation and it has antioxidant properties, ginseng may help to prevent the development and growth of certain cancers.

One particularly important benefit of ginseng is that it appears to promote energy and fight fatigue. Some of the compounds found in ginseng help to lower oxidative stress, which will result in higher levels of energy. People who regularly use ginseng are known to experience less mental and physical fatigue than those people who do not use ginseng. It is also beneficial in lowering blood sugar which is another way it works to boost your levels of energy.

Milk thistle – This herbal remedy already has a long history of being used for medicinal purposes. It has long been used to protect the liver from environmental toxins, treat and prevent cancer, promote the production of breast milk, and treat disorders of the gallbladder and the liver.

This herb is regularly used to compliment therapies used for the treatment of liver cancer, hepatitis, and alcoholic and non-alcoholic liver disease. People who have any form of liver disease will benefit from taking milk thistle extract. It is thought that the milk thistle reduces the damage to the liver that is caused by free radicals that your liver produces when it metabolizes substances that are toxic.

Milk thistle has also been used to treat neurological conditions like Parkinson's disease and Alzheimer's disease. It helps to prevent brain function decline because of its antioxidant and anti-inflammatory properties. Milk thistle seems to be beneficial in reducing plaques in the brain, little clusters of protein that interfere with normal brain function.

In laboratory experiments, it appears that milk thistle can help to prevent progressive bone loss that is the main cause of osteoporosis. Milk thistle may enhance the effectiveness of cancer treatments. It also appears to be effective in treating acne and preventing the scarring that can come with excess facial acne. And it can help to lower blood sugar levels in people who have type 2 diabetes.

Chapter 5: Herbals to Prevent Disease

Humans have sought out remedies for illnesses and ailments within their environment since the beginning of time. Even today, traditional systems of medicine are built partially upon methods for preventing disease. The use of herbal medicines is an ancient tradition, and recent developments in traditional medicine have reignited interest in herbal medicines for the prevention of disease. Here are some of the most well-known herbs that are used for the prevention of disease.

Holy Basil – This is not basic basil. It is not the same as the sweet basil that is found in the cabinet in your kitchen, the basil that you use to flavor your marinara sauce. This herb comes from a leafy green plant that is also known as tulsi and is found in Southeast Asia. Holy basil has long been used in Indian medicine for treating conditions from ringworms to diseases of the eye. From the seeds to the leaves, holy basil is considered to be a natural tonic for your spirit, mind, and body. The entire plant is recommended for human use for its therapeutic value. It also has a high nutritional value, since it contains chlorophyll, iron, zinc, calcium, and vitamins A and C.

Different parts of holy basil will treat different ailments of the body:

- Make an essential oil from the leaves for insect bites
- Use an alcohol extract for eye disease and stomach ulcers
- Pills and ointments of this herb are used to treat eczema
- Parts of the whole plant will treat vomiting, nausea, and diarrhea
- Mix the seeds and leaves with black pepper to treat malaria
- The fresh flowers from the plant treat bronchitis

All of the parts of the holy basil plant act as an adaptogen, which is a natural substance that will help promote mental balance and will help your body react better to stressful situations. Holy basil has properties that will assist with emotional, infectious, physical, and chemical stress. When dealing with physical stress, holy basil is known to lower stress levels in loud environments, lead to less tissue damage, and enhance your metabolism. Studies of holy basil on both animals and humans saw incidences of reduced exhaustion, forgetfulness, sleep problems, sexual problems, and stress.

Ayurvedic medicine recommends using the leaves to make a tea and drinking it daily since it is caffeine-free. It will foster a sense of well-being, relaxation, and clear thought. Holy basil has anti-anxiety and antidepressant properties that will help people to feel less depressed stressed, and anxious.

Holy basil is used to boost the strength and speed of healing wounds. Holy basil has all of the properties of an effective medication since it is analgesic, anti-inflammatory, antifungal, antiviral, and antibacterial. For prevention purposes, holy basil is good for the following conditions:

- Holy basil increases the natural defenses of your stomach by extending the life of mucus cells, increasing the mucus cells, increasing the secretion of mucus, and decreasing the production of stomach acid. Mucus in the stomach helps protect the lining of the stomach against the attack of stomach acid.
- Holy basil has antioxidant and anti-inflammatory properties, which makes it a natural defense against joint pain and inflammation. It is particularly effective against fibromyalgia and arthritis.
- Holy basil helps to raise good cholesterol and lower bad cholesterol, which will help to prevent cardiovascular disease. This herb will also assist with weight loss by targeting metabolic stress.
- Holy basil will keep your blood sugar lower, which will help to prevent the physical symptoms that signal the onset of diabetes like hypertension, insulin resistance, high cholesterol, and weight gain.

You can easily add holy basil to your daily routine by taking a supplement that is available in capsule or pill form. You can also use the dried powder of the leaf or flowers, or the fresh flowers or leaves, to make a tea for daily drinking. Put two to three teaspoons of holy basil in one cup of boiling water and let this tea steep for five minutes.

Cumin – Cumin is a spice used in recipes from Asia and the Mediterranean. Besides being an ingredient in curry, tamales, and chili, it has been used for hundreds of years in traditional medicine. Cumin assists with preventing diabetes, treating cancer, boils, skin disorders, anemia, bronchitis, asthma, and insomnia, aiding in digestion, and improving immunity.

- Cumin has anti-inflammatory properties that will help to lower and prevent inflammation.
- Components in cumin help to reduce symptoms of withdrawal and addictive behavior, so it can help to prevent dependence on chemicals that lead to addictions.
- Cumin is used to season foods, and it has antimicrobial properties that can help to reduce the risk of people suffering from the effects of food-borne infections. Compounds in cumin will reduce the growth of certain types of infectious funguses and food-borne bacteria. After it is digested, cumin releases a compound that has

antibiotic properties, and it can also reduce the resistance of some bacteria to medications.

- Concentrated supplements of cumin may help to prevent excess weight gain.

- Cumin supplements have been shown to decrease triglycerides in the blood, which will lead to a healthier heart. Cumin used in regular cooking or taken as a supplement can help to keep blood triglycerides lowered.

- Cumin works to prevent the damaging effects of the substances in the blood of a diabetic person that attack the small blood vessels, nerves, kidneys, and eyes. The compound work to control blood sugar levels, and when taken regularly, can lead to overall lower blood sugar levels, which may help to prevent the onset of diabetes.

- Cumin possesses many different plant compounds known as alkaloids, flavonoids, phenols, and terpenes that carry many benefits for your health. The compounds function as antioxidants in the body, and they work to reduce the damaging effects of free radicals in your body. A free radical is an electron that has split off from its cell and is in search of another free radical electron to pair with since they like to be in pairs. They will readily attach themselves to healthy cells and cause inflammation and damage to the DNA of the cell.

- Cumin is a good source of your daily needs of iron. One teaspoon has 1.4 milligrams of iron, which is seventeen and one-half percent of the amount that you are recommended to have daily for good health. Regular ingestion of cumin will help to prevent iron deficiency anemia, especially in children and women.

- Cumin is most traditionally used for improving the process of digestion. It can help to increase the activity of your digestive enzymes, which will work to speed up your metabolism. And cumin speeds up the release of bile from your liver, and bile works to digest certain nutrients and fat in your gut. Using cumin regularly can also help to ease the symptoms of irritable bowel syndrome, and regular use of cumin may help to prevent digestive diseases.

Cumin is easy to add into your regular daily routine by just adding it to your food. Cumin is a warm spice with a hint of a lemony flavor and slightly bitter undertones. It brings a spicy, nutty flavor to foods when it is added in. Cumin, as a spice, can be added to almost any dish.

Oregano – Most people think of oregano as the herb for pizza. Besides being used to enhance or improve the flavor of foods, oregano also has many benefits for your health. It is full of minerals and vitamins, especially vitamins E, C, and A, as well as the minerals niacin, manganese, copper, potassium, calcium, iron, magnesium, and zinc. Oregano has long been used to improve the health of the heart, kill intestinal parasites, relieve the cramps of menstruation, combat the virus that causes flu and the common cold, and relieve the pressure of nasal congestion.

- Oregano is very easy to add to your daily diet. Besides being the perfect herb for use on pizzas and in pasta dishes, it is also delicious when added into stews, soups, chili, and salads. It also works well in salad dressing and fresh pesto. Oregano is available as an oil, or as a fresh or dried herb, so it is simple to use every day.

- Oregano is loaded with antioxidants that can reduce inflammation and fight the ravages of free radicals. Since chronic inflammation can lead to the development of many diseases like autoimmune conditions, diabetes, and heart disease, decreasing or eliminating chronic inflammation will help to prevent these diseases from developing.

- Oregano has components that will protect against viruses, so using oregano regularly will help to prevent people from contracting viruses. Two compounds in oregano, thymol, and carvacrol, have been shown to inactivate many different forms of viruses like herpes simplex and norovirus.

- Oregano is loaded with antioxidants that can aid in the prevention of cancer and also assists with neutralizing free radicals, which are known to contribute to the development of cancer.

- Oregano has compounds that carry potent antibacterial properties. The essential oil of oregano will help to kill several strains of bacteria that cause infection.

- Oregano is full of antioxidants that work to kill off the free radicals in the body and fight the damage that they cause. Free radicals building up in the body have been linked to the development of chronic diseases like heart disease and cancer. Using oregano regularly will help to prevent the buildup of chemicals in the body that will cause chronic illnesses.

Oregano is a flavorful addition to everyday recipes that also carry impressive benefits for your health. The antioxidants will empower your body and give it the strength to fight off viruses and bacteria, help to relieve chronic inflammation, and possibly inhibit or reduce the growth of cancer cells.

Sage – This powerful healer has been used since the Middle Ages. Sage comes from an evergreen shrub that has purple or blue flowers and woody stems. Sage, as a medicine, was initially used to boost female fertility and treat snakebite. Sage is also known to aid digestion, help with the management of diabetes, treat acne, psoriasis, and eczema, assist with the development of stronger bones, strengthen the immune system, eliminate cognitive disorders, and boost memory and information recall. The flavor of sage is earthy, and the aroma is strong, so it is usually used in small amounts. It is available in dried or fresh forms or as oil.

- Sage is very easy to add to your daily diet. You can mix it with eggs to make an omelet, chop it up and stir it into tomato sauce, blend it into stuffing mixes, and sprinkle it on stews and soups as a garnish. It is also an excellent seasoning for roasted vegetables and roasted meats.

- Sage has compounds that may fight off the formation of wrinkles, help to build strong bones, and relieve diarrhea.

- Sage extracts stimulate the death of cancer cells and also work to suppress their growth.

- Sage tea can help to reduce levels of cholesterol in the blood to prevent damage to the arteries and the heart.

- Sage is loaded with antioxidants that will help to stop the breakdown of certain chemical messengers in the brain. It can also improve performance on cognitive abilities like reasoning, problem-solving, and memory.

- Sage extract can help to reduce levels of sugar in the blood, which will help to prevent diabetes. It will also help to prevent insulin resistance and sensitivity.

- Sage has compounds that mimic estrogen, and it is often used to reduce the symptoms of menopause like irritability, excessive sweating, and hot flashes.

- Sage helps to fight off dental plaque with its microbial properties. A mouthwash made of sage kills the bacteria that are known to cause dental cavities. Sage can also be used to treat and prevent mouth ulcers, infected gums, dental abscesses, and throat infections.

- Sage has more than one hundred sixty polyphenols that act as antioxidants that work to neutralize the free radicals that will cause damage in the cells in your body. Many of the compounds found in sage help to improve memory and brain function and lower the risk of cancer.

- Sage is loaded with minerals and vitamins. In just one teaspoon of sage, you will find manganese, calcium, vitamin B, iron, and vitamin K.

Sage is safe to use on a regular basis with no known side effects. It is delicious in foods and also makes a wonderful tea.

Nutmeg – This spice grows on an evergreen tree, and it is native to Indonesia. Cuisines all around the world make use of nutmeg, and it is prized for its slightly sweet and delicate flavor. It is well known to have an impact on health in several ways because it contains a large number of organic compounds, minerals, and vitamins. Nutmeg will also provide you with copper, magnesium, folate, vitamin B6, thiamin, manganese, and dietary fiber. Nutmeg will help to lower blood pressure, combat insomnia, kill bacteria in the mouth, promote good digestion, enhance the health of your brain, relieve pain and inflammation, and detoxify the body.

- Nutmeg is not only a versatile spice, but it is also delicious. In the kitchen, it is often paired with cloves, cinnamon, and cardamom. This spice is usually used to flavor custards, fruit salads, breads, cookies, cakes, and pies. It is also a good addition to meat and vegetable dishes, and it can be sprinkled on top of smoothies, lattes, chai tea, hot chocolate, and apple cider to add a delicious spiciness to the drink.

- Nutmeg might be beneficial for controlling blood sugar, high cholesterol, and high triglycerides. It might also help to improve your moods since it has an anti-depressant effect in humans.

- Nutmeg can be potentially helpful against harmful strains of bacteria because it has antibacterial properties. It is especially effective against gum inflammation and cavities. And the anti-bacterial properties of nutmeg may help to lessen the effects of E.coli bacteria.

- Nutmeg may lower the levels of inflammation in your

body because of its anti-inflammatory properties. Since chronic inflammation is linked to the development of arthritis, diabetes, and heart disease, reducing or eliminating chronic inflammation may help t prevent the development of these and more chronic diseases.

- Nutmeg is loaded with plant compounds that have antioxidant properties in your body. The antioxidants in nutmeg work to fight the free radicals in your body that cause damage to your cells. These free radicals are known to cause cancer, heart disease, and degenerative diseases of the nervous system.

Many kitchens all over the world have the spice known as nutmeg in one of their cabinets. It is a popular ingredient in many different recipes. And besides being an amazing spice for consumption, nutmeg is also loaded with antioxidant and anti-inflammatory properties.

Cinnamon – This spice used to be used as barter in the world of trade. Cinnamon was also used medicinally for thousands of years. Besides being an extremely tasty spice, it can also fight off fungal infections and bacteria, may protect against certain cancers, might work to cut the risk of heart disease, can help to lower blood sugar levels, and is anti-inflammatory and antioxidant.

- Cinnamon may be an effective treatment against HIV-1, which is the most common strain of HIV that is present in the human body.

- Cinnamon has active compounds that can help to fight infections of the respiratory tract. This spice may also effectively reduce bad breath and help prevent tooth decay.

- Cinnamon shows promise in the treatment and prevention of certain types of cancer.

- Cinnamon contains compounds that seem to inhibit the buildup of proteins in the brain that may cause Parkinson's disease and Alzheimer's disease.

- Cinnamon is useful for lowering blood sugar and may help to prevent diabetes. It has the ability to decrease the amount of glucose that can enter your bloodstream after eating. Cinnamon interferes with several of the digestive enzymes that slow down the digestion of carbohydrates, which leads to less sugar entering your bloodstream.

- Cinnamon has the ability to dramatically reduce insulin resistance, so it helps to improve the body's ability to move blood glucose into the cells where it can be used for energy. And reducing insulin resistance will also help to reduce or prevent diabetes and metabolic syndrome.

- Cinnamon works to reduce your risk of developing heart disease by reducing triglycerides and cholesterol levels in the blood.

- Cinnamon has properties that help to reduce inflammation in the body, which will help to repair damage to your tissues and also help to fight infection.
- Cinnamon has antioxidants that will help to protect the body from the damage caused by free radicals.

Of all the spices in use today, cinnamon is one of the most delicious and also the healthiest. Cinnamon can reduce inflammation, lower the risk factors that lead to heart disease, and lower blood sugar levels.

Garlic – This herb is anti-fungal, antibacterial, and antiviral. Garlic can also relieve nasal congestion and coughing, treat earaches and toothaches, fight inflammation and cancer, and detoxify the body.

- Garlic is a delicious addition to any diet and very easy to use. Garlic is particularly tasty in sauces and soups. It is available in oil, extract, powder, paste, and whole cloves.
- Garlic used daily can help to keep women's bones strong and healthy after menopause.
- Garlic consumption can help detoxify the body after exposure to heavy metals.

- Garlic has enhanced athletic performance for centuries. It can enhance the capacity to work and reduce fatigue.

- Garlic can help you to live longer by fighting infectious diseases and strengthening the immune system.

- Garlic has powerful antioxidants that fight the free radicals in your body that might lead to the development of dementia and Alzheimer's disease.

- Garlic can lower the risk of developing heart disease by improving cholesterol levels in the blood.

- Garlic contains compounds that are known to prevent strokes and heart attacks by reducing blood pressure levels.

- Garlic supplements work to boost the strength and function of the immune system, which can significantly reduce the number of days someone might suffer the effects of cold or flu.

- Garlic has very few calories but is very nutritious. It contains vitamin B1, iron, phosphorus, potassium, copper, calcium, fiber, selenium, vitamin C and B6, and manganese. And there is only one gram of carbohydrates in one clove of garlic.

Garlic is closely related to leeks, shallots, and onions. The delicious taste and strong smell make it a popular ingredient in many recipes. Garlic has long been highly prized for its medicinal properties.

Rosemary – This herb is native to the Mediterranean regions and is thought to enhance brain function and memory. Rosemary has anti-aging properties, helps to detoxify the body, is an anti-inflammatory, works to stimulate the flow of blood in the body, relieves body aches and stomach upsets improves mood and has antibacterial properties.

- Rosemary extract can promote heart health and treat indigestion.
- Rosemary has compounds that might help to slow the progression of eye diseases that are related to aging.
- Rosemary may protect against degenerative diseases like Alzheimer's
  disease by preventing the premature death of brain cells.
- Rosemary reduces inflammation in the part of the brain that controls mood, leaving people feeling happier. It can also work to boost the powers of your memory.
- Rosemary may help to prevent or reduce the symptoms of diabetes by lowering blood sugar levels.
- Rosemary contains compounds that are antimicrobial and anti- inflammatory. While it is often used to preserve perishable food, it can also

help to heal wounds and fight infection.

- Rosemary oil rubbed on the scalp may help to eliminate dandruff while it stimulates hair growth.
- Rosemary has properties that make it an excellent pain reliever. It can also be beneficial for improving circulation.
- Rosemary can relieve and reduce stiffness, pain, and swelling by reducing inflammation in tissues. It can be particularly effective against rheumatoid arthritis.

Rosemary is particularly easy to use, especially in the form of essential oil. It is especially useful when used for inhaling. Diluted with a carrier oil, it is effective against skin rashes and for rubbing sore muscles.

Ginger – Ginger has been used for centuries to treat and prevent diseases. Ginger can help fight infections, protect against Alzheimer's disease and improve brain function, prevents high cholesterol levels, and treats and prevents nausea.

- Ginger can prevent the spread of infections with its antimicrobial properties.
- Ginger can prevent chronic inflammation and oxidative stress that will accelerate the process of aging.
- Ginger may help to prevent cancer by helping to

control the growth of abnormal cells.

- Ginger can help to prevent strokes and heart attacks by lowering cholesterol levels and blood sugar levels.
- Ginger can treat and prevent chronic indigestion by speeding up the rate at which food is emptied from the stomach.
- Ginger can help to prevent degeneration of the joints in the body by preventing inflammation of the joints.
- Ginger can prevent soreness and muscle pain that occurs after intense exercise because of its anti-inflammatory properties.
- Ginger can treat and prevent nausea associated with pregnancy, seasickness, and chemotherapy.

For its medicinal properties as well as in recipes, ginger has been used for centuries. It can be used as a juice, oil, powder, dried, or fresh. Its medicinal properties include its antioxidant and anti-inflammatory compounds.

Turmeric – This herb might easily be the most powerful herb on the planet. It contains several compounds that have medicinal properties. Turmeric is one of the herbs that are most frequently mentioned and discussed in science.

- Turmeric prevents blood clotting and helps to keep the blood thin and flowing freely, which will help to prevent blood clots.

- Turmeric will help to prevent depression by helping to control the hormones that cause it.

- Turmeric can prevent the effects of arthritis and inflammation due to its anti-inflammatory properties.

- Turmeric can help to prevent diabetes by reversing insulin resistance and lowering blood sugar.

- Turmeric may prevent indigestion and other ailments of the digestive tract by feeding the good bacteria in the gut.

- Turmeric can reduce the risk of developing heart disease by regulating blood clotting and blood pressure.

Turmeric and the most active compound it has that is known as curcumin, has the potential to prevent cancer, Alzheimer's disease, and heart disease. It has many other health benefits that have been used for centuries.

Spices and herbs are part of the culture and history of the world. Many spices and herbs contain plant compounds that are powerful enough to heal our bodies, ease our aches and pains, and even prevent serious diseases. Mummies in ancient

Egypt were preserved with spices and herbs. Spices and herbs were used as barter for trading. Today people use many of the spices and herbs that have been used since the beginning of recorded history to prevent disease, spices, and herbs like nutmeg, cloves, ginger, cinnamon, cumin, and turmeric. All of these herbs and spices can be used on a regular basis to prevent disease.

Chapter 6: Growing Your Own Herbs

Herbs are one of the most natural things that you can grow. They grow well with some form of light, a bit of water, and some fertilizer now and then. Gardening with herbs has become much more popular in recent years as people are putting more emphasis on food that is nutritious, delicious, and fresh. Recipes made with herbs grown at home will always taste better. Herbs are among the easiest plants to grow, and they grow well with little effort.

If you are gardening in a small space, you can make an herb garden out of a collection of pots on the windowsill in the kitchen or in the corner of the patio. There are no rules that are set in stone for the growing of herbs. Any guidelines you will need to follow will depend on the actual herb that you are planning to grow. If you are growing annual herbs like dill, coriander, chervil, and basil, then they will want to be located where there is full sunshine. Herbs that are native to the Mediterranean region, like oregano and lavender, love warm temperatures and full sun. Moist settings like wooded areas are perfect for shade-loving herbs like sweet woodruff and mint.

With the exception of a few herbs that prefer to be grown in the shade, all herbs share four growing conditions that they all have in common:

- To keep the herb plants full, give them regular harvesting and trimming. Some people do not like to prune the plants in their gardens, preferring to leave the plants to grow at their own will. But if you are growing the herbs in order to use them, then they will need regular trimming and pruning. Herbs that are not treated to regular trimming, herbs that are not cut for use, will more quickly go to seed, and they will also grow very tall and unmanageable. Even the perennial woody herbs like sage, lavender, and rosemary will have less dead, weak wood, and they will grow fuller and healthier if they are treated to regular pruning.

- Herbs like to enjoy regular drinks of water, but they also like to have good drainage. There are very few plants that like to live in damp soil or like to have their roots continually damp. Roots that are constantly wet will eventually rot. Even if the roots don't rot, leaving them wet all the time will invite disease and weaken the structure of the plant. This is even more important when you are planning on using the leaves, stems, or roots of the herb plant. And it is not a good idea to go the other way either. While the herbs that are native to the Mediterranean area, like lavender, thyme, oregano, or rosemary, are more tolerant to drought conditions, they will not grow well if they do not receive the proper amount of water. Pay attention to the plant as it will tell you when it is thirsty.

- Sunshine and light are very important for the health of the herb. The essential oil levels, and the flavor and the fragrance of the herbs, are intensified by good soil and warm sunshine. Herbs need at least six hours of full light every day.

- The soil should be healthy but not too rich. Herbs prefer a soil that is more lean than rich, so do not be too overgenerous with fertilizers. Most herbs do not do well in rich soil. Flowering herbs need plenty of water and rich soil so that they will develop bountiful flowers. The herbs will not develop good flavor and intense scent if they are grown in soil that is too rich.

Once your herbs are growing, you will need to water them when the top inch of soil feels dry when you poke your finger in it. Do not water the herbs too much, and let the water drain away rather than sit in a pool around the herb. When it is time to harvest your herbs just cut off about one-third of the branches when the plant grows to be at least eight to ten inches tall. Cut the branch off close to the intersection with a leaf so that the herb will be stimulated to grow more.

Growing Herbs in Containers

Many herbs will grow well in a container. If you grow your herbs in pots, then you will be able to suit the potting soil to the particular herb. Every plant prefers its own mixture of nutrients, and growing plants in pots make this easier to do. Pots can be moved around easily in the yard, kitchen, or deck; so that you can create beautiful plant displays or just keeps the herbs close to the kitchen door for easy access to fresh herbs when you are cooking.

The containers you use can be as conventional or as wild as you prefer them to be. Feel free to use containers that you have lying around the house or the garage, or use those quirky items you found at garage sales and thrift stores. Use galvanized tubs, concrete urns, plastic buckets, or terracotta pots. Grow one herb per pot or group several together.

While most herbs will grow well in containers, it may be necessary to give some of them their own pot, since some, like mint, like to overwhelm and take over its neighbors. And knowing your herbs will allow you to put herbs together in pots that like the same conditions for growing, like a particular nutrient mix or amount of water.

Whatever kind of container you choose to use, the container will need holes in the bottom to drain out the excess water. If the pot does not come with drain holes, then you will need to drill some in. Then place a few pieces of broken pottery over the drain holes to keep the soil in while the water drains out. Mix a few small pebbles, like aquarium rocks, in with the soil so that it will drain well. Before setting your herbs in the dirt, lay them together so that you can choose the best possible arrangement. When you are ready to plant your herbs, fill the pot halfway with soil and begin setting the herb plants in, adding more soil around and under their roots as needed. Press the soil down gently, but don't pack it in the pot. If the dirt is too firm, the roots will have trouble spreading.

Once you have all of the herbs planted in the pot, water them until the water begins to drain out of the drain holes in the bottom of the pot. You might want to write the names of the herbs on wooden sticks and stake them in the dirt near the plant if you are new to growing herbs and might forget which herb is which.

Your herbs plants will now grow on their own with very little maintenance, but there are a few things that you can do to endure that your harvest is bountiful. Water your herbs to the needs of the individual herbs. Aromatic herbs with smaller leaves, like thyme or rosemary, require minimal watering. Herbs with fleshy leaves like basil and parsley need to be watered more often. Use a liquid fertilizer every two to three weeks to keep your herbs well-fed without overfeeding them.

Herbs like to be trimmed and harvested regularly, so don't be afraid to enjoy the fruits of your labors.

Seven Best Herbs for Growing in Pots

Lemon Balm – This member of the mint family likes to take over the available space just like mint does, so it does particularly well growing in containers. This hardy perennial likes plenty of water, so it will develop its best flavor. The green leaves of a healthy plant will be glossy, and they will taste and smell like lemons. You can use the leaves in marinades, lemonade, teas, and salads.

Parsley – This herb comes in two varieties, flat-leaf and curly-leaf, and both grow well in a container. Parsley not only grows well, but it also looks good. This herb wants regular feeding and moisture, and it will grow from the beginning of spring until the end of autumn.

Mint – There is no one herb that can be called mint. You can grow spearmint, strawberry mint, mojito mint, chocolate mint, and peppermint, just to name a few. The leaves of the mint plant can be used in teas, fruit salads, and summer drinks. Mint plants like a rich soil with ample watering.

Thyme – This herb is one of the best herbs that you can grow in a container. Besides being low maintenance, it really looks good when it is planted. Since thyme is resistant to drought, it does not want to be watered very often.

Rosemary – The needle-like foliage on this woody shrub makes a welcome addition to chicken dishes and roasted potatoes, among other things. While most varieties of rosemary grow upward, some are vine-like and will cascade over the sides of the container. And while the rosemary like constant moisture, it does not like to have its roots too wet, so do not overwater this herb.

Oregano – This herb likes to run wild, so it is best to keep it in a container. Trim the leaves off as often as possible and use them in your bruschetta, homemade pizzas, and tomato-based sauces.

Basil – This herb is an annual that loves the warm weather and loves to be in any kind of container. As long as the soil drains well and the light is strong, basil will grow well for you. If your basil starts to make flowers pinch them off, a basil plant that is flowering looks nice, but it will drain the entire flavor out of the leaves.

Growing Herbs From Seeds

An herb garden is the perfect kind of garden to grow if you are a beginner gardener or if you live in an area that does not have much space. Growing your herbs from seeds is not as difficult to do as you might think it is. All you need to grow herbs from seeds are the seeds themselves with some potting soil, some small containers, and a little bit of sunlight.

You will want to look for some important things when you are buying your seeds, and all of this information will be available on the packet of seeds. You will first want to know how deep you will need to plant the seeds. You will next want to know the thinning space and the seed spacing. You might initially plant your sees six inches apart and then later thin them out so that they are twelve inches apart. Since not every seed will germinate, you will always plant more seeds than the amount of plants that you will want to grow. It is also good to know which month is the best month to plant your seeds, and this will depend on what area of the country that you live in. You will need to know the mature size of the herb since this will help you determine the layout of your garden or how large the container will need to be. The packet will also tell you about how long it will take the seeds to germinate and how long it will be before you can expect to make your first harvest. The information that you will find on the packet of seeds will give you all the information that you need to plan your garden properly.

The soil, or growing medium, that you will want to use is very important when you are growing your herbs from seeds. There are different purposes for different types of soil, and you will need to know the difference, so you will know which soil to use when:

- To start your seeds indoors, you will want to use a seed starting mix.
- Whether you transplant your herbs to containers for indoor or outdoor growing or you transplant them to a garden, you will want to use potting mix.
- Herbs planted in pots for setting outdoors will use either potting mix or potting soil. The difference between the two is the amount of perlite or compost mixed into the soil. Smaller sized or indoor pots will use a lighter mix of soil. Outdoor plants or larger planters will need a heavier potting soil.
- Garden soil is another type of soil mix, and this will be worked into the ground when you transplant your herbs into an outdoor garden space.
- Do not bring plain dirt from the ground indoors or anywhere else to use in your pots. Ground dirt should remain on the ground.

When you are growing herbs from seed indoors, you will not use dirt or soil. You will use a mixture called a seed starting mix, which is a very fine mixture that will allow the tender roots to be able to grow and develop. Seed starting mix does not come with the extra fertilizers that mixes meant for full-grown plants will have.

The seed has all of the nutrients that it will need to start its growth cycle, so the seedling will not require any extra nutrients until it has grown two sets of real leaves. And do not use moisture control potting soil mix to start your seeds, as it might retain more moisture than the seed needs, and it might cause the seed to rot. In fact, when growing herbs, or any other plant, from seed, it is a good idea for the soil to become a bit dry so that the young roots will stretch and seek water.

Seven Herbs to Grow from Seeds

Cilantro/Coriander – Many people don't know that these two herbs come from the same plant, but the leaves are the cilantro, and the seeds are the coriander. Cilantro prefers cooler temperatures in the beginning of its growth, so start it in the early spring. It does not like to be disturbed for transplanting, so grow the seeds in some type of growing plug that can be transplanted with the seedling. Lay one to two inches of soil over the seeds, water them gently, and then the seedling to keep them four inches apart when they have two sets of leaves.

This herb will mature within four weeks, so if you sow new cilantro every three weeks, then you will have a constant supply of cilantro and coriander. The seeds will germinate in ten to fifteen days and grow to be one to two feet tall. Cilantro prefers at least six hours of light every day.

Parsley – Soak the parsley seeds in warm water for twenty-four hours before planting them because parsley seeds take forever to germinate, and this will help to speed up the process. Cover the seeds with a one-eighth inch of soil and keep the soil moist. If you are transplanting the seedling outdoors, wait until all danger of frost has passed and plant the parsley eight inches apart. The plants will need to be watered regularly without letting the soil dry out completely. Parsley will grow to be twelve to eighteen inches tall. The seeds will take fourteen to twenty- eight days to germinate, and the plant likes to have at least six hours of light every day.

Chives – This herb will grow in clumps like spiky grass. Begin with the seeds indoors at least six weeks before the normal time of the last frost in your area. Chives like to grow in well-drained soil, and since they grow in clumps, there is no need to thin them out to give them space. When the plants are young, they will want a lot of water. When the plant has reached six inches in height, take the leaves on the outside of the clump and cut them almost to the level of the soil as this will encourage the chives to grow faster. Chives grow to be ten to twelve inches tall, and they like four to six hours of light each day. The seeds will germinate in ten to twenty days.

Sage – This perennial, shrubby shaped herb grows well indoors from seeds. Start your seeds indoors four to six weeks before the last frost in your area. Sage likes to grow in loamy or sandy soil that is well-drained. Water the plants often until they are fully developed; after that, the plant is very much drought resistant. Let the plant grow to its full height before attempting to harvest any of the leaves.

Sage will grow to be twenty-four inches tall and likes six hours of light every day. The seeds will germinate in ten to twenty days.

Oregano – This herb germinates its seeds in seven to fourteen days, grows to be twenty-four inches tall, and likes to have at least six hours of light every day. Start your oregano seeds indoors about six to eight weeks before the average days of the last frost in your area. Since oregano seeds need some light to germinate, you will only sprinkle them on the surface of the soil; you will not cover them. After sprinkling the seeds make the soil moist without disturbing the seeds. Oregano likes soil with a loam mixture that drains easily. When the plant has grown to six inches, start cutting off stems and leaves as needs, as this will encourage growth on the plant.

Thyme – The seeds of this herb also do not like to be covered, so drop them on the potting mix and moisten the soil lightly without disturbing the seeds. Thyme takes ten to fifteen days to germinate and likes at least six hours of light daily. It will grow to be six to twelve inches tall. Only feed thyme plants when you transplant the seedling because this herb does not require a lot of nutrients to grow well. It likes a dry soil that is slightly sandy in its composition, and once it has begun growing, it is relatively drought resistant.

Basil – This annual herb grows to be twenty-four inches tall, likes six hours of light every day, and will germinate in five to ten days. Start your basil seeds indoors about six to eight weeks before the last frost for your area. Always keep the soil that basil is planted in evenly moist, and it prefers to grow in a loamy soil that is well-drained and full of organic matter. You want the plant to spread its leaves out, so pinch off the top stem of the plant to encourage broader growth.

It is easy to grow herbs, either from seeds or from cuttings off other plants. You can grow your herbs either indoors or outdoors. And once the plant is established, the herb will require very little maintenance and will give you a generous amount of harvest with very little work.

Chapter 7: Medicinal Herbs

While most people are familiar with the herbs that they use for cooking, they are not necessarily familiar with the use of herbs for medicinal purposes. Here are some of the herbs that are used medicinally.

Most Commonly Used Medicinal Herbs for Prevention of Illnesses

Aloe Vera – The juices from the leaves of the Aloe Vera plant are used for making lotions, creams, and gels for healing numerous ailments of the skin. This herb has properties that are antiviral, antifungal, and antibacterial, which make it an excellent wound healer. It has the ability to regrow skin after a burn, and Aloe Vera has anti-inflammatory properties and stimulates the production of collagen, a key ingredient in maintaining healthy skin. Aloe Vera gel will help to prevent wrinkles. The juice of the Aloe Vera plant prevents high triglycerides in the blood and helps to prevent digestive ailments.

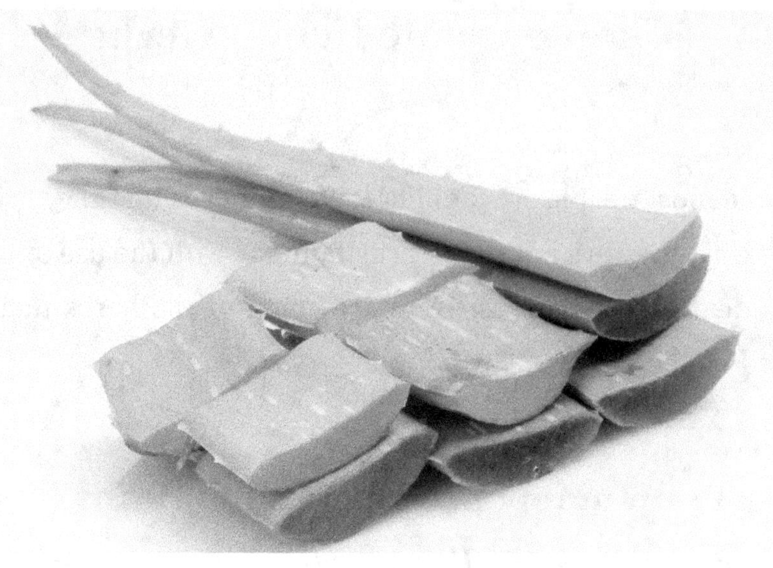

Anise Seed – This herb has therapeutic powers that are often used in herbal remedies to kill the germs of the virus while it helps to move the virus out of the chest and sinuses. It works to prevent and relieve bloating and gas for centuries.

Arnica – This alpine herb has a long, rich history of medicinal use. It is used as both a cream and oil. If the cream is used directly after an injury to the muscle, it will greatly relieve the injury to the muscle. It is also effective in reducing joint pain, bruising, and swelling, which is due to fractures. It has anti-inflammatory properties that help to prevent inflammation while it works to move fluids out of swollen areas and healing blood flow into the affected area.

Basil – This member of the mint family helps to settle the stomach and improve appetite. It is also used to treat headaches and common colds. Basil, when used regularly, will help to relieve inflammation that can lead to heart disease.

Bilberry – While this herb will help to relieve the bruising and swelling from black eyes, it is better known for its abilities to prevent gout by lowering the levels of uric acid in the blood. Extracts from the bilberry plant will lower high blood pressure and high cholesterol and can be effective in treating or preventing diabetes.

Black Cohosh – This herbal remedy is a wonderful cough reliever. But it is mainly known for treating the symptoms that are associated with menopause by mimicking estrogen without the adverse effects that excess estrogen can have on the woman's body.

Calendula – This herb has anti-inflammatory and antibacterial properties that make it the perfect herb for treating and preventing all types of skin issues and irritations, as well as other infected areas. Made into a facial wash, it treats acne and dry skin, preventing the inflammation and rashes that often come with these two conditions. Used as a tea, it will treat all sorts of mouth and throat issues like infected gums, sore throat, and mouth sores.

Cardamom – This herb has antispasmodic properties, which make it an excellent treatment for any type of digestive upset like IBS, indigestion, nausea, and even morning sickness that is caused by pregnancy. It will clear the congested lungs and sinuses people get with allergies, flu, and the common cold. Taken regularly as a tea, it will kill the bacteria that are responsible for bad breath and strengthen the digestive system.

Celery Seed – This herb will not only reduce your dependence on salt when cooking, but it will also decrease the uric acid content in your blood. At the same time, it also decreases the excessive buildup of water, which makes it an effective method for preventing arthritis and gout.

Chamomile – This is the first herb of choice for many home prevention recipes and treatment remedies. Chamomile has antibacterial and anti-inflammatory properties and is effective in the digestive system and the nervous system. When taken as a cup of tea, the antispasmodic properties will calm tense muscles and help to prevent muscle aches, pains, and spasms.

Cilantro – This herb will detoxify your system and work to prevent digestive upsets.

Cinnamon – Just a little bit of this spice will spread energy and warmth throughout the body. People with type 2 diabetes can rely on cinnamon to lower their blood sugar levels, and taken regularly; cinnamon may help to prevent diabetes. It is also an effective remedy for flu and the common cold because of its antibacterial properties. Used regularly in foods can help to prevent diseases of the mouth.

Clove oil – The antibacterial agents in clove oil will help to prevent viruses and colds when you use it to clean surfaces. It is often used for toothache and other dental pains because it is an effective antiseptic and analgesic treatment for mouth issues. It is also effective in easing the pain of arthritis in the joints and muscle aches. Clove will ease nausea and other digestive upsets, and taken regularly; it will help to strengthen the digestive system and prevent further upsets.

Comfrey – This marvelous herb is known as one of the best herbs of all time for its healing and preventive properties. It relieves the inflammation and pain that is associated with arthritis and injuries to the body. People will find relief, especially for the conditions of osteoarthritis and rheumatoid arthritis.

Ointments and salves made from comfrey can treat or prevent almost any skin irritation like insect bites, flea bites, lacerations, abrasions, skin ulcers, and minor burns. Comfrey will speed the healing of wounds and eczema. When used as a compress on sprains, fractures, and bruises, it will speed healing because one of the compounds in this herb is known to increase the production of new cells inside and outside the body. In a tea, it will treat coughs and sore throats, and is effective in treating and preventing ulcers of the stomach.

Dandelion Root – This herb will help the body to get rid of undesirable skin bacteria. This herb also supports the function of the liver and works to stimulate digestion. Giving support to the liver is extremely important because this organ is the one that is most in charge of ridding the body of toxins. It will help to normalize and regulate the production and use of hormones in the body, particularly the feminine hormones. It has natural properties for diuretic and laxative use, so it will help to rid the body of the buildup of toxic substances.
Taken regularly, dandelion root will help to prevent the buildup of toxins and excess weight.

Dill – This unique and very familiar smell can automatically make most people's mouths begin to water. Just like the herb cilantro, both the seeds and the leaves of dill can be used for cooking and for their medicinal properties. Dill will ease nausea and relieve bloating and gas. When dill is used to make tea, it will promote the beginning of a woman's monthly cycle and will also help to promote an increase in the production of breast milk.

Echinacea – All varieties of echinacea have compounds that will naturally improve the function of your immune system.

When taken at the first indication of gum inflammation or flu or the onset of the common cold, echinacea proves to be an effective therapeutic agent. It is most effective when used regularly for the prevention of viruses and bacterial infections. It will relieve the itching that is associated with hives and insect bites when it is used as a wash.

Eucalyptus – Anyone who has ever used any kind of rub for relieving congestion is familiar with the smell of eucalyptus. It is an effective remedy for colds because it is known to relieve bronchial congestion, clear out clogged passages in the sinuses, and encourage freer breathing. Used as an essential oil in a carrier oil, a few drops will relieve the pain of arthritis and stiff joints and muscles. When taken as a tea, it will not only take away the aggravating symptoms of a cold or allergy, but it will also help to relax you.

Fennel Seed – As a digestive aid, this herb will relieve the symptoms of bloating, gas, and abdominal cramping. When they are added to vegetables that would normally produce gas and bloating in the abdomen, the fennel seeds will work to prevent these complaints. When the seeds are made into a tea, they will soothe the hacking, dry cough of bronchitis because a compound in fennel seeds helps to make the cough more productive by loosening the congestion in the chest. When fennel seed tea is consumed fifteen to thirty minutes before mealtime, it will work to prevent overeating and can help to prevent excessive weight gain.

Garlic – Cooking with fresh garlic on a regular basis will help to prevent stomach and colorectal cancers. It will relieve the pain of skin irritations and burns when it is applied directly to the skin in a poultice. And adding the cloves to your recipes will help to lower blood sugar and blood cholesterol, thereby assisting with the reduction of the risk of developing heart disease, arthritis, and diabetes.

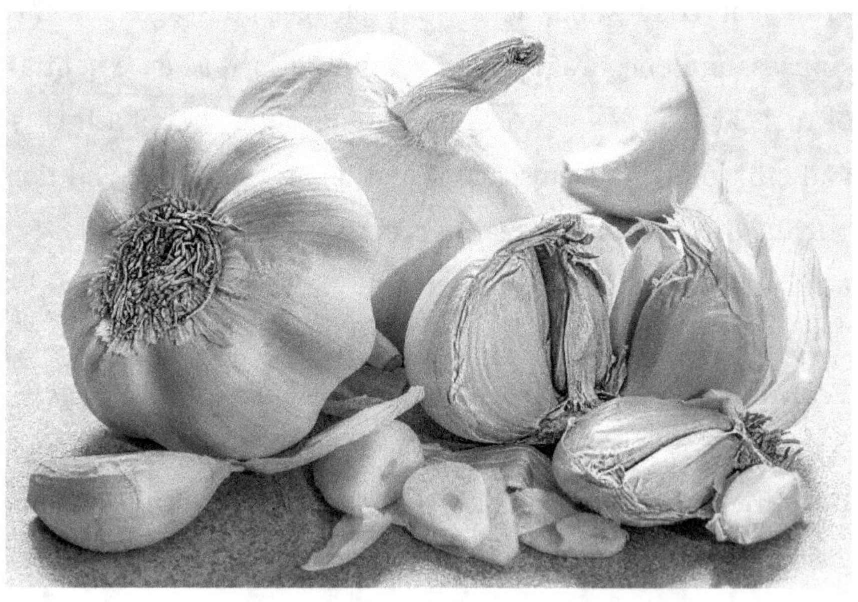

Ginger Root – This herb has been used for centuries for its medicinal properties. It will safely and effectively treat a wide range of health problems, from arthritis to simple nausea. One of the most impressive features of ginger is that it can be added to any other herbal remedy to improve the taste of that herbal remedy without altering the basic formula or its health benefits. Ginger works to thin the blood, making it flow through the body easier and helping to prevent the buildup of plaque and lowering cholesterol. Tea made from the ginger root will improve the health of the digestive system and will help to prevent nausea, particularly nausea that is commonly experienced after surgery or during chemotherapy treatments.

Ginseng Root – This is another herb that has been used medicinally since the early days of recorded medicinal treatments. This herb will strengthen the immune system when used regularly. It can help to relieve the severity of the symptoms of cold and flu and may help to prevent these viruses from attacking humans. It can also help to lower the levels of sugar in the blood, which will work to prevent diabetes. It is also used to help boost physical endurance and improve moods.

Hawthorn Berry – Since medieval times, this herb has been used as an effective tonic for strengthening the heart. This herb decreases the levels of lactic acid in the blood, which is the waste product that comes from physical exertion and causes pain and swelling in the muscles, especially in the heart muscles. It will also improve energy metabolism and oxygenation in the heart and help to dilate the arteries of the heart. Hawthorn makes the job the heart does easier because it relaxes the blood vessels, making it easier for the heart to pump efficiently. This herb will also help to cure sore throats, ease digestive upsets, and help you to sleep better.

Hibiscus – This herb has long been known for its beautiful flowers, but it also has amazing medicinal properties. Since it is loaded with vitamin C is a natural antioxidant. It is also a very gentle laxative and diuretic, helping to prevent the buildup of toxins in the body. Regularly drinking hibiscus tea will lower blood pressure and help to avoid the chronic conditions of the cardiovascular system that are associated with high blood pressure.

Horseradish Root – This herb is used for medicinal purposes because of its antibiotic properties. When taken for the common cold, it will soothe a sore throat, loosen sinus and chest congestion, and stimulate the nerves in the area to help the body to heal itself. It also stimulates the flow of blood throughout the body, so when it is used in a compress, it improves the circulation and warmth to cold, stiff joints and muscles. When ingested regularly, it is an effective prevention for rheumatism and gout.

Lavender -- This herb is pretty to look at, and it is loaded with medicinal properties. Used as a tea or in an herbal bath, it can restore poor circulation and aid in restful sleep. It works to improve blood circulation and to lower high blood pressure. A few drops of the essential oil in a carrier oil can be applied to the forehead to ease a headache or to any joint to ease pain and swelling. It also has analgesic properties when used against nerve pain, sore muscles, and arthritis. It can help to prevent muscle aches and pain.

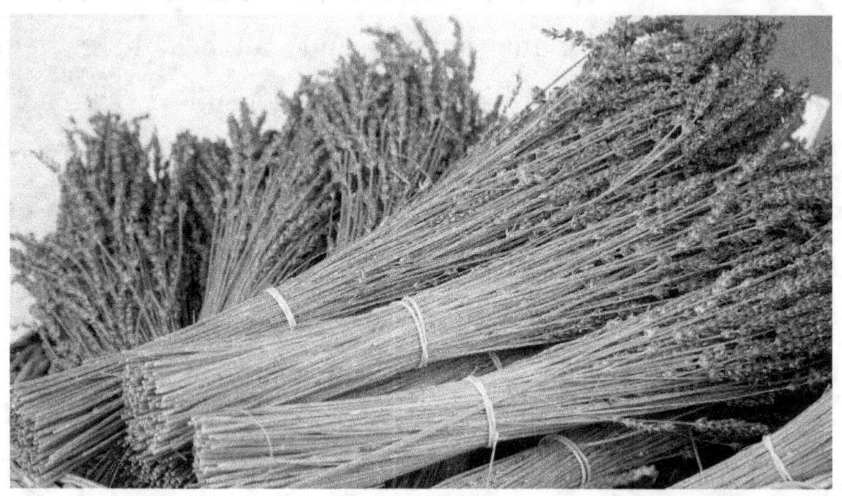

Lemon Balm – This herb is a valuable medicinal plant, as well as being useful for aromatherapy. The calming properties of lemon balm can help to relieve mild depression, headache, and it works to soothe tense nerves. It has valuable antiviral and antibacterial properties, which make it an excellent remedy in the fight against cold and flu. Regular use of lemon balm will help to strengthen the immune system and work to repel viruses and bacteria.

Lemongrass – This herb is well known in the Far East and the Middle East for its medicinal properties. It works to flush toxins from the body and will also stimulate the body to digest fats faster and easier. When the essential oil is blended with a carrier oil, it is useful for relieving skin irritations.

Mint – The uplifting aroma of this tea is enough to soothe frazzled nerves. When the tea is consumed, it will relieve stomach and abdominal spasms and can help to prevent bloating and gas after a heavy meal is consumed. This herb also assists with relieving and preventing digestive upsets such as irritable bowel syndrome. It is also an excellent herb for fighting the symptoms of a cold because of its ability to ease breathing and loosen congestion. It will also soothe sore throats, fever, muscle aches, and congestion.

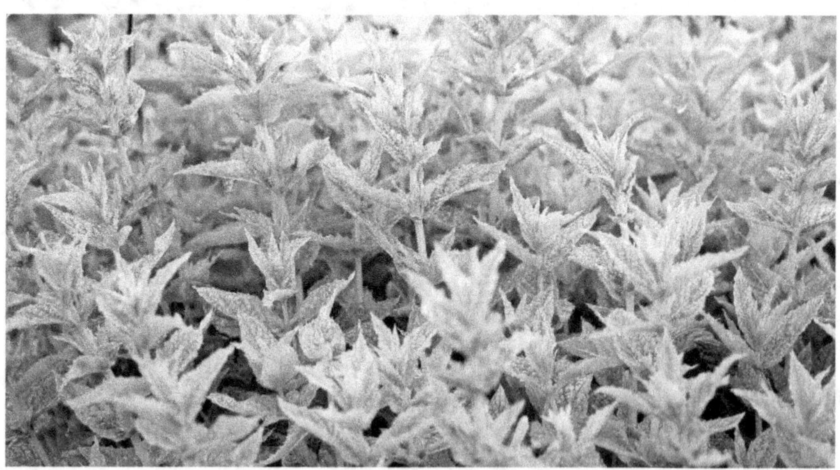

Mustard – This herb will work to warm and stimulate the digestive system. The oil of the mustard seed is known to stimulate the circulation of blood throughout the entire body.

Its antibacterial properties kill germs and viruses while it works to relieve congestion in the lungs and sinuses. When used a poultice on the chest, it will assist even more in the removal of congestion, and it will also ease the pain of inflamed joints.

Oregano – This herb is not just the primary ingredient in pizza sauce, but it is also an herb that is ranked first among the culinary herbs because of its powers and a natural antioxidant. Most of the medicinal properties that oregano has are due to its compounds that make it an antioxidant, antibacterial, and anti- inflammatory agent. By relieving inflammation in the body, oregano can help to prevent stroke, heart disease, and many types of cancer. It also helps to lower blood sugar, which makes it an effective weapon in preventing diabetes. And regular consumption of oregano tea will work to strengthen the digestive system.

Pine – The needles of the pine tree are actually an herb, and they are prized for their ability to reduce pain in people who suffer from sore muscles, aches and pains, and arthritis. The oil of pine needles is often used in cold and cough medicines and in fluids for the vaporizer to relieve colds and coughs. The oil also has analgesic and decongestant properties. When the oil is mixed with a carrier oil and massaged on the body, it can help to reduce the pain and swelling of gout and arthritis. It is also effective in removing and preventing stiffness in the joints when it is used in an herbal bath.

Pumpkin Seed – Besides being good to eat either raw or toasted, the pumpkin seed and its oil are an effective treatment for healing injuries to the skin like wounds and burns. The pumpkin seed is best used when it is cold because heating the pumpkin seeds destroys the properties that make it a healthy herb. The seeds are a great source of fatty acids, which will help to prevent excess body weight from accumulating, and they are good for the health of your heart. They are effective in treating bladder infections and worms and parasites that attack the digestive system. Regular consumption of pumpkin seeds and the use of its oil on salads will help to prevent ailments of the digestive system that are caused by harmful bacteria.

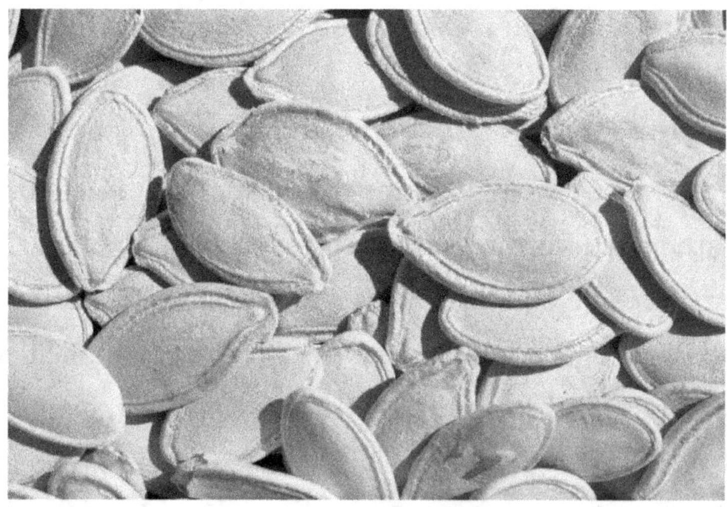

Rose – This beautiful flower has long been grown in gardens in European monasteries and used for its medicinal properties. The petals of the rose plant have astringent properties and can be used as an effective skin wash to clean cuts and scrapes and stop the bleeding. Rose oil and rose petals are commonly used in skincare preparations, notably in formulas designed for the face because they are a gentle yet powerful way to kill the bacteria that cause skin ailments and irritations. And when the petals are used in the bath, they will have the same cleansing effect on the skin as well as helping to relax the mind and body.

Rosemary – This herb is useful for preventing ailments of the central nervous system and the circulatory system. It helps regulate blood pressure. The oil of rosemary can relieve the symptoms of neuralgia, sciatica, arthritis, and sprains. The essential oils that are found in the leaves will block the chemical histamine, which is the main culprit that causes allergies and asthma attacks. Use it in boiling water to make steam that will clear congestion and restore free breathing. Rosemary can be consumed daily in the form of oils and vinegar, with many excellent health benefits for the bod.

Sage – This herb has long been believed to be the key to a long and healthy life. Sage is remarkable for easing indigestion and other digestive upsets. It is also a remedy for fever and cold when taken as a tea, especially if lemon is added. Sage also has astringent and antibacterial properties that make it an excellent remedy for sore gums and sore throats, as well as killing the bacteria that cause all kinds of diseases of the mouth and throat. Sage will also work to heal irritations of the skin and to aid in strengthening concentration and memory.

Sesame – The herbs and oil of this plant have been used for hundreds of years for their medicinal properties. Sesame seeds will help to promote the healthy function of the liver. The compounds in the seeds will also relieve constipation, high cholesterol, and high blood pressure. The oil is often used in Asian cuisines. It is considered to be a stable carrier oil for home cosmetic use and for aromatherapy. And the oil has naturally active levels of the vitamins A and E, which make it beneficial to the skin.

Skullcap – This herb comes in many different varieties, and only the ones that contain the compound scutellarin are used in herbal medicine. Skullcap has been used as a natural sedative and a tonic for the nerves for centuries. This herb is to relieve nerve pain, anxiety, and nervous tension. In Traditional Chinese medicine, skullcap is used to relieve fevers, swelling, thick mucus, and irritability.

St. John's Wort – This herb has a demonstrated ability to relieve anxiety and mild depression, as well as acting as a natural tonic for the entire nervous system. The tea has long been used to stop the problems of incontinence, particularly during sleep, in both adults and children. It is recommended to be used with all types of illnesses from diarrhea, worms, bladder problems, and heart problems. It is also an effective skin aid, especially when used on herpes lesions, because it is both analgesic and anti-inflammatory. When the essential oil of St. John's Wort is blended with a carrier oil, it is an effective rub for muscle aches, fibromyalgia, arthritis, and sciatica.

Sunflower – The seeds of the sunflower and the oil that is extracted from them are the parts of the sunflower that are most often used for medicinal purposes.

The seeds carry the powerful antioxidant known as melatonin, which aids in restful sleep. It makes a good carrier oil for essential oils and can be used to soften the skin and relieve skin irritations.

Tea Tree Oil – This has a broad range of antifungal and antimicrobial properties, which make it a natural addition to herbal remedies. It will take care of almost any skin irritation from flea or mosquito bites to fungus and bacterial infections. Tea Tree Oil can be used as an effective remedy for acne. Its antiviral properties make it a natural remedy for treating infections of the sinuses and respiratory system as well as working to stimulate the immune system in the body. Take a drop or two daily to help prevent viruses and bacterial infections.

Thyme – This is one of the best herbs to relieve the symptoms of coughs and colds. It is a natural antitussive, so it will calm the spasms of coughing. And it is a natural expectorant so it will clear congestion from the sinuses and the lungs.

Drinking thyme tea will flush toxins from the body, lower fevers, and promote restful sleep. It is also an effective treatment for infections of the skin because of its antiseptic properties.

Turmeric – This herb has been scientifically confirmed to be one of the primary anti-inflammatory herbs. Two of its active ingredients will relieve inflammation as well or better than many over-the-counter anti-inflammatories. This is also why the regular consumption of this herb is linked to a reduced risk of developing Alzheimer's disease, cataracts, and certain cancers. It will also work to relieve the skin irritation of psoriasis and the pain of rheumatoid arthritis. This herb is also effective when used against diseases of the mouth. It has antimicrobial, antioxidant, and anti-inflammatory properties.

Valerian Root – This herb is probably the most widely used herbal sedative available. It will help you to relax in the presence of pain and will also work to relieve your nervous anxiety and insomnia. While it is a potent relaxer and sleep aid, it is not addictive. And not only will this herb help you to fall asleep faster, but it will also help you to sleep better. It will also relieve muscle aches and calm coughs.

White Willow Bark – This herb has been used for thousands of years to combat pain, inflammation, and fever. One of the compounds in common aspirin is derived from a compound that is found in white willow bark. The beneficial effects of this herb in the body last longer than aspirin but take effect more slowly, so they cause less gastrointestinal upsets than aspirin does. And it is highly effective when used along with other herbs in formulas that promote weight loss. You can make a solution of this herb to aid in the healing of cuts, burns, and scrapes, and it can also be used as an antibacterial and soothing mouth wash.

Witch Hazel – The essential oil from this herb makes a mildly astringent and soothing lotion for skin irritations. Since it is gentle and mild, it is one of the home remedies most widely in use even today. It is an excellent all-around treatment for insect bites, scalds, burns, abrasions, and many other ailments of the skin. Witch hazel is also one of the primary ingredients in the treatment of varicose veins. When used on the skin of the face, it will reduce the size of pores, puffiness of the skin, and under-eye bags while it works to gently but effectively cleanse the skin.

Other Medicinal Herbs

Bee Balm (also known as wild bergamot) – This herb has antimicrobial properties, so it is often used to treat viruses like the flu and the common cold. It also has soothing abilities, so it is also used to treat nausea, bloating, and indigestion.

Coltsfoot – This flower is used to make an herbal tea that will relieve the symptoms of fever, gout, flu, sore throat, and respiratory infections.

Elderflowers – This flower from the Elder plant will help to alleviate the inflammation of swollen sinuses caused by bronchitis, flu, the common cold, and sinusitis.

Evening Primrose – The oil extracted from this herb will help to alleviate skin irritations.

Feverfew – This herb has been used for centuries as a tea to relieve fevers, and it is now most commonly used to treat arthritis and prevent migraine headaches.

Flax Seed – The oil from the seeds and the seeds themselves have anti- inflammatory and antibacterial properties.

Ginkgo – The extract of the leaf of this herb will treat a variety of illnesses from ringing in the ears, fatigue, bronchitis, and asthma.

Goldenseal – This herb is often used in the treatment of skin irritations, diarrhea, and irritations of the eye. It is used to make an antiseptic preparation.

Lady's Mantle – This herb is strictly for the ladies to relieve the pains and aches associated with being female.

Marsh Mallow Root – This root has an anti-inflammatory effect and is particularly useful against skin irritations like dermatitis, eczema, and rashes.

Milk Thistle – This herb will reduce the rate of growth of cancer cells as well as reducing high cholesterol and aiding in the health of the liver.

Mullein – Also known as the flannel leaf plant, this herb will lessen the symptoms of pneumonia, tonsillitis, and bronchitis.

Osha Root – This root of the osha plant has compounds that make it excellent for the support of your immune system. It is also an expectorant, decongestant, diuretic, antiviral, antimicrobial, antibacterial, and anti-inflammatory.

Pennyroyal – This herb is made into a tea to ease indigestion and headaches.

Poppy – The petals of the poppy are known to help induce sleep and to soothe coughs associated with whooping cough and bronchitis.

Raspberry Leaf – This herb is loaded with minerals and vitamins, as well as antioxidants.

Red Clover – This herb will alleviate the cough that accompanies bronchitis, asthma, whooping cough, the flu, and the common cold. It will also lower high cholesterol and help to prevent indigestion and cancer.

Sorrell – This herb is a diuretic, as well as known to reduce fevers.

Vervain – This herb is widely used for its ability to ease breathing associated with colds and flu.

White Clover – When the blossoms are used to make tea, it is used for eyewash. A tincture mixed with cream can be used as an ointment to treat gout.

Yarrow – This herb will help to relieve skin problems like abrasions, cuts, and wounds.

Chapter 8: Recipes for Using Medicinal Herbs

You can easily buy blend or herbal teas in most grocery stores and big-box

retailers, but they will be full of chemicals that you don't want and won't have enough of the beneficial ingredients that you do want, since most of them are made with artificial flavors and not real herbs. Making tea from real herbs is not difficult, and some people find the practice to be rather enjoyable. Look for a reputable herb shop where you can buy fresh and dried herbs if you are not growing your own herbs. Don't overlook local growers and farmer's markets and stands. When you make the herbal tea, it is okay to make extra and store it in a glass jar in a dark place. The teas will stay fresh for three or four days.

You will want to use at least one teaspoon of herbs for every eight ounces of tea that you are making. Experiment with making your own blends. Most of the best herbal tea blends follow a specific basic structure. This is also true for herbal medicinal teas, since you would mix these teas and then add them to the medicinal herb if you are making your own blends.

- **Flowering flavor** -- Most basic blends will include some type of flowery flavor. Some of the more common choices are wild rose petals, calendula petals, dandelion petals, chamomile flowers, and violet flowers. You will use one part* of this herb.

- **Placeholder flavor** -- The next flavor that you add will be the flavor that ties all of the other ingredients together. This flavor will also lend strength to the tea in case you serve it over ice. You will want to add in two parts of this herb, and dried nettles or the leaves of the red raspberry work very well.

- **Fruity flavor** – A naturally sweet herb or a fruity herb is the next herb that you will add, and you will use one part of this herb. Hibiscus flowers or dried rosehip is a good choice for this part.

- **Cooling flavor** – Add one part of any of the mint herbs or borage to add a refreshing component to your tea.

A part is that item measured as a fraction, no matter what measure you are using. You can use a tablespoon or a one-cup measure or a pound, but one part is one part. So if you are using tablespoons, you would use three tablespoons for three parts of the herb.

Here are a few recipes for different herbal teas.

Elderberry Tea

Ingredients:

- Two whole cloves
- Two cardamom pods
- One cinnamon stick
- One tablespoon of dried elderberries
- Two cups of water

Directions:

1. Drop all of the ingredients into a pot and simmer the mixture for thirty minutes.
2. Strain the mixture carefully into a cup and sweeten the tea with the sweetener of your choice.

Immune Support Tea

Ingredients:

- One-fourth cup of echinacea
- One-fourth cup of astragalus
- One-fourth cup of rose hips
- One-fourth cup of chamomile
- One-fourth cup of elderberries

Directions:

1. Mix all of the herbs together into a glass jar and store until you want to make tea.
2. When it is time to drink the tea, just add one or two teaspoons into a cup of boiling water and give the tea time to steep for at least ten minutes before straining and drinking.

Warming Ginger Tea

Ingredients:

- One-half teaspoon of honey
- One-fourth cup of lemon juice
- One piece of ginger root, one inch long and minced

Directions:

1. Put the three ingredients into a cup for serving and pour very hot, but not boiling, water over them.
2. Let the ingredients steep for five to ten minutes.
3. The more extended period of time that the tea steeps, the stronger it will become.
4. Strain the ginger out before drinking the tea if you prefer.

Sore Throat Remedy Tea

Ingredients:

- One one-liter glass jar with a lid
- Boiling water to fill the jar
- Eight to ten fresh leaves of sage

Directions:

1. Drop the leaves into the glass jar and pour the boiling water over them, filling the jar almost all of the way to the top.
2. Put the lid tightly on the jar and let the tea steep for ten to fifteen minutes.
3. You can use this tea to gargle when your throat is scratchy or inflamed.
4. If you are using this therapeutically, then you will want to drink at least three cups every day.
5. Feel free to flavor the tea with sweetener and/or mint leaves.

Thyme Tea

Ingredients:

- Two teaspoons of lemon juice
- One-fourth cup of fresh thyme sprigs
- One pint-sized glass jar
- Freshly boiled water

Directions:

1. Place the sprigs of thyme into the glass jar and then fill the jar with the freshly boiled water.
2. Steep the thyme in the water for ten minutes.
3. Strain out the thyme leaves and stir in the lemon juice.
4. Add sweetener if you prefer.
5. This tea will ease cold and cough symptoms.

Green Tea with Rose Hips Tea

Ingredients:

- Four teaspoons of maple syrup
- One pinch of cayenne pepper
- Two tablespoons of rose hips
- One-fourth cup of lemon juice
- One tablespoon of fresh green tea
- One to two cups of water

Directions:

1. Boil the water and place the rose hips and the green tea in a cup for serving.
2. Pour the boiling water over the items in the serving cup and let them steep for ten minutes.
3. Strain out the rosehips and the green tea leaves if desired and stir in the lemon juice, maple syrup, and cayenne pepper.

<u>Cayenne Tea</u>

Ingredients:

- One cup of boiled water
- One teaspoon of honey
- One tablespoon of lemon juice
- One-eighth teaspoon of cayenne pepper

Directions:

1. Put the cayenne pepper into a mug and pour the boiling water over it.
2. Then stir in the honey and the lemon juice and enjoy.
3. You can use more cayenne pepper if you like your drink a bit spicier.

<u>Respiratory Support Tea</u>

Ingredients:

- Two parts of rose hips
- One part of lemon balm
- One part of coltsfoot, either flowers or leaves or both
- One part of mullein
- One part of osha root
- One part of marshmallow root

Directions:

1. Add three cups of water to a saucepot and put the osha roots and the marshmallow root in the water.
2. Boil this mixture and then let it simmer for ten to fifteen minutes.
3. Then add in the remainder of the ingredients and let it steep for ten minutes more.
4. Strain out the herbs and drink three to four cups of this daily to prevent the respiratory ailments caused by viruses.

Cold Care Tea

Ingredients:

- One part of elderflowers
- One part of hibiscus flowers
- One part of sage leaves
- One part of calendula flowers
- One quart-size glass jar with a lid
- Two to three cups of boiling water

Directions:

1. Drop the herbs into the glass quart jar and then cover them with the boiling water, filling the jar until it is almost full.
2. Put the lid tightly on the jar and let the tea steep for ten minutes.
3. When you are ready to drink the tea strain out the herbs and add a little honey or sweetener if it is desired.

Autumn Tea Tonic

Ingredients:

- One part of ginger root, dried
- One part of rose hips
- Two parts of red clover
- Two parts of dandelion
- Two parts of mullein
- Three parts of lemon balm
- Three parts of spearmint
- Four parts of nettle
- Gallon glass jar

Directions:

1. Put all of the ingredients together in the glass jar with a lid and fasten the lid on securely.
2. Shake the jar gently to mix all of the ingredients together well.
3. When you are ready to drink the tea, pour four cups of boiling water over the tea blend in the glass jar and let it steep for at least fifteen minutes, but if you can leave it undisturbed for up to eight hours the tea will be more potent and beneficial.
4. Strain out the herbs and add in a little sweetener if you like.
5. Drink this tea at least once daily to prevent viruses and bacterial infections that come with autumn and winter.

Lavender Tea

Ingredients:

- Three tablespoons of lavender flowers, either fresh or dried
- One-half cup of fresh lemon balm
- Three cups of hot water
- Serving mug

Directions:

1. Pour boiling water over the lavender and the fresh lemon balm in the mug.
2. Cover the mug with something to keep the steam in and let the tea steep for five minutes.
3. Strain the tea to remove the herbs and add in sweetener if you want to.

Peppermint Tea

Ingredients:

- Eight ounces of boiling water
- One teaspoon of honey
- One teaspoon of dried peppermint

Directions:

1. Put the peppermint and the honey into a serving mug and pour the boiling water over them.
2. Steep the tea for ten minutes and drink it hot or pour it over ice.

After Dinner Digestion Tea

Ingredients:

- One-eighth part of dried licorice root
- One part of spearmint leaves
- One sprinkle of fennel seeds
- One sprinkle of ground cloves
- One glass jar with a lid

Directions:

1. Blend all of the ingredients together in the glass jar, put the lid on securely, and shake the jar gently.
2. When you want to enjoy, the tea put one tablespoon into a serving mug and pour boiling water over the herbs, and let the tea steep for five minutes.

Calming Marshmallow Rose Tea

Ingredients:

- One cinnamon stick
- One-half part of ground cinnamon powder
- Two parts of holy basil
- Two parts of rose hips
- Three parts of marshmallow root
- One quart-size glass jar with a lid

Directions:

1. Blend all of the herbs together in the glass jar and put the lid on securely.
2. Until you want to drink the tea store the sealed jar in a cool, dark place.
3. Then put one-fourth to one-half cup of the herb mix into a tea kettle and add in hot water.
4. Steep the herbs in the tea for ten minutes and then strain out the herbs and add in sweetener if you desire.

Lemon Tisane

Ingredients:

- One part of chamomile
- One part of grated lemon peel
- One part of lemon balm
- Three parts of lemongrass
- Quart size glass jar with lid

Directions:

1. Place all of the herbs into the glass jar and securely fasten the lid.
2. Shake the jar gently to completely mix all of the herbs.
3. Store the glass jar in a cool, dark place until you are ready to drink the tea.
4. Then add one teaspoon of the herb mix to a serving mug and add in boiling water.
5. Let the tea steep for ten minutes with a plate over the mug to keep the steam in.

Herbal Tea for Women

Ingredients:

- One part yarrow flowers
- One part white clover
- One part Lady's mantle
- One part raspberry leaves
- One quart-sized glass jar with lid

Directions:

1. Drop the herbs into the glass jar and secure the lid.
2. Shake the jar gently to mix the herbs together.
3. When you are ready to drink the tea, place one tablespoon of herbs into a serving mug and pour fresh boiling water over the herbs.
4. Place a plate over the mug to keep the steam in and let the tea steep for five minutes.
5. Strain the herbs out and sip the tea while relaxing.

Astragalus Immune Support Tea

Ingredients:

- One and one-half quarts of water
- Five whole cloves
- Two tablespoons ground allspice
- Two cardamom pods
- One teaspoon of peppercorns
- One tablespoon of ground cinnamon
- Two tablespoons of dried orange peel
- Two tablespoons of ginger root
- Ten slices of licorice root
- Two tablespoons of astragalus root

Directions:

1. Drop all of the ingredients into a medium-sized saucepan and let the mixture boil.
2. Then let the mixture simmer on low for one hour and strain out the herbs.
3. Serve with sweetener if you desire to.

Conclusion

Thank you for making it through to the end of *Herb Antivirals*, let's hope it was informative and able to provide you with all of the tools that you will need to achieve your goals whatever they may be.

The next step is for you to begin using your own herbs for treating your ailments and preventing viral illnesses that can bring your life to a standstill. When you have become comfortable experimenting with different herbs, you will be well on your way to achieving a healthy lifestyle with the assistance of herbal remedies.

There are so many herbs available for use in the world today, and many of them have been around since man first started experimenting with different herbs. The world of herbs is an amazing world just waiting for you to unlock all of its potential for your health and wellness.

Finally, if you found this book useful in any way, a review on Amazon is always appreciated!